EAT AND GROW SLENDER

LELORD KORDEL

EAT AND GROW SLENDER

The *Sure* Way To Get Slim—and *Stay* Slim

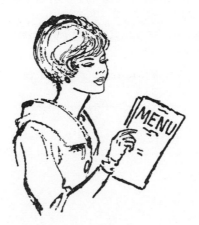

THE WORLD PUBLISHING COMPANY

CLEVELAND AND NEW YORK

Published by *The World Publishing Company*
2231 West 110th Street, Cleveland 2, Ohio

Published simultaneously in Canada by
Nelson, Foster & Scott Ltd.

Library of Congress Catalog Card Number: 62-15711

FIRST EDITION

Drawings by Polly Bolian

Contents

CONTENTS

EAT AND GROW SLENDER

1

Are You Fatter Than You Think?

ONCE THERE WAS a time when you dreamed of yourself as slender, glamorous, and alluring. Or maybe it wasn't just a dream. Let's suppose that you *were* slim and stream-lined—once upon a time.

How long ago was that? Two years ago? Five? Ten? Or more than you care to count?

Pounds are no respecters of age, wealth, or position. They can accumulate on anyone, young or old, rich or poor, any time, anywhere.

Their favorite trick is to creep up on you gradually when you're not looking. There you are, just sitting quietly minding your own business—eating your fudge cake alamode—and those sneaky pounds start settling on you behind your back.

Also in front, in the middle, and all around you.

Then one day you take a good long look at yourself in a full-length mirror and think, "Is that a *shadow* of a dou-ble chin? A *suspicion* of a fat and flabby stomach? Hips that are—to put it mildly—hippy?"

When that happens, what do you do about it? Ignore

the extra pounds and hope that they'll go away all by themselves? Buy a dress a size larger and believe that nobody will notice? "Me—gaining weight? What an idea! Look how loose my clothes are!"

Or do you protest angrily, "This can't happen to *me!*"

It has happened, though. To you, personally.

And unfortunately pounds can't be ignored away. To my knowledge, nobody has yet been able to coax them away, either. They refuse to be bluffed or scared away, and even exercise can't chase them away to any noticeable extent.

But they can be eaten away!

Please stop right here and turn down a page in your memory. Remember that I said *eaten away*—not *starved away.*

You *can* eat to beat the pounds. But going on a diet which is deficient in the essential proteins, vitamins, and minerals is not the way to do it. Malnutrition can give you a puffy tummy just as surely as overeating will. A semi-starvation diet will age your skin, wreck your nerves, and ruin your disposition—not to mention your health, beauty, vitality, and glamour.

The pounds you lose will be your own.

But so will the fatigue, the flabbiness, the haggard, hungry look, the dull eyes, sagging, wrinkled skin, and the vital tissues that have been destroyed in the process.

Whether you call them crash diets, miracle diets, or starvation diets, they are not worth the sacrifice. *Certainly not when there is a sure way to eat and grow thin, glamorous, and healthy all at the same time.*

Not long ago a young woman came to me and asked for help in planning some reducing menus for her husband. Like most men, she said, he couldn't be bothered counting calories, and he'd heard about a book which assured him that he didn't have to.

"But when he eats all the fats he wants," she told me, "he gains so much that he simply can't believe it and thinks the scales are wrong. He won't do anything about it, so I'm going to have to. I want to learn how to give him low-calorie meals that will reduce him and won't leave him feeling hungry."

"He *can* forget about calories," I said, "but only if a basic eating pattern is followed that automatically includes the *right* type of calories, which most emphatically *do* count, if you value your health, youthfulness, and general appearance."

Dr. Jean Mayer of the Harvard School of Public Health is world-famous for his studies on the causes of obesity. He bristled at the thought of calories not counting, when he made this comment:

"The idea has no basis in theory, will not work in practice, and is positively dangerous."

The trim Dr. Mayer confirmed my own teachings when he said, "The idea that the kinds of food you eat and not the amount you eat is important . . . is contrary to the findings of scientific studies."

But to get back to the young woman in question for whose husband I worked out a series of high-protein, forget-about-calories, fool-the-appetite meals which included plenty of bulky vegetables and fruits to give him a feeling of satiety at low calorie cost:

"Of course I've never had to bother with reducing," she said rather smugly. "My weight is exactly average for my height and age."

"What do you mean by average?" I asked.

"Well—just *average,* that's what I mean by average. My

weight is perfectly normal according to the tables of weights that I've seen in my doctor's office and in magazines. I'm five feet, five inches tall, twenty-nine years old—"

She hesitated for a moment, and I thought to myself, "Oscar Wilde said that a woman who'll tell her age will tell anything. But she says she's twenty-nine years old, and no doubt she is—perhaps has been for two or three years. It doesn't matter. Whatever age a woman is doesn't matter at all. Any age can be a charming one for the slender, vital woman."

Aloud I merely said, "Yes? Go on."

Her voice took on a triumphant note as she said, "And I weigh exactly 129 pounds!"

My reaction was a big disappointment to her. "Just as I thought," I said. "Let's see, you have a small frame. Small wrists, small bones, and narrow shoulders. You're about eleven pounds overweight, and should start reducing right along with your husband."

"I can't believe I'm overweight!" she said. "But even if you're right about it, ten or eleven pounds are certainly no cause for alarm."

"You think not?" I asked.

Dr. Frederick J. Stare of Harvard University's Nutrition Department says that even ten pounds over normal weight can mean that you run the risk of dying five or ten years sooner than you otherwise might.

"You're in the alarm zone," according to Dr. Stare, "if you're ten pounds overweight. "We're reasonably certain that normal weight gives you the best chance of living out your expected life span."

And what is normal weight?

If you've considered yourself normal or average in weight by outmoded standards, then you are anywhere from ten to twenty pounds overweight, give or take a few

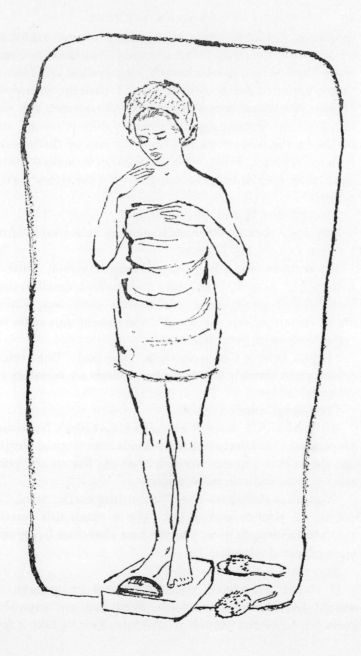

pounds, depending on whether you have a small, medium, or large frame.

The old weight tables are as out of date as high-button shoes, and should be thrown away. They no longer serve any purpose except to fool you about your best weight for health, beauty, and longevity. Such a misconception can be decidedly dangerous.

Now, don't get angry with *me*.

It isn't my fault that the tables have been literally turned on you, proving that instead of being normal in weight many of us may be fatter than we think.

The new weight tables were compiled by the men who have a big stake in your weight. They have a financial interest in your waistline, since they know it's your life line. They are the insurance men.

Your lack of health and vigor hits them where it hurts the most—in their bank account. So naturally one of their most fervent desires is for you to lose weight—and live longer.

The Metropolitan Life Insurance Company, for the first time in almost twenty years, has completely over-hauled its own widely used tables of desirable weights for men and women.

It was a tremendous and very commendable task, which began with a study by the Society of Actuaries of nearly 5,000,000—that's right, five million!—insured persons. Here are some of the things that their study revealed:

1. Nearly half of all men and women over 30 years of age are 20 per cent or more above their best weight.

2. Both sexes gain in weight as the years go by. Men put on most of the extra pounds between 20 and 40, and women start a slow (but steady!) gain after 35.

3. From a health standpoint, women bear the extra

weight a good deal better than men. (But how it does deglamorize and age you in appearance!)

4. If you're 20 pounds over your best weight, as indicated on the new Metropolitan Life tables, your mortality rate is 10 per cent above average. If you're 25 pounds overweight, the rate is 25 per cent higher. And if—heaven forbid!—you're 50 pounds above average, your chances of living as long as your slender friends are almost non-existent. Your mortality rate is 50 to 75 per cent higher than theirs.

5. Some of the ailments which, combined with overweight, will hasten death, are diabetes, certain digestive disorders, and, of course, heart disease.

6. The danger of high blood pressure increases when the patient is overweight to such an extent that the insurance companies are considering raising the premium rates on such cases.

7. The old weight tables allowed for an increase in weight as you grow older. *The new ones do not.* Let birthdays come and go. On you they'll look good if you find your best weight for your height and bone structure, then work to achieve and sustain that weight for the rest of your life, which should be a long and happy one.

Forget the old weight tables with their misleading figures, and concentrate on these new ones, for both men and women, which are included in the next chapter.

But don't just sit there and concentrate. At least not for too long.

You know perfectly well that sitting isn't going to make you lose weight, and neither will the most intense concentration, without a little action on your part. In fact, you'd have to do six hours of mental work to burn up the 50 calories that you get in one cup of coffee with a teaspoon of sugar and a tablespoon of cream in it! (Black coffee or tea, without sugar—*no calories*.)

"All right," you say, "you've convinced me that I really should lose ten, fifteen, or maybe twenty pounds if I want to look and feel my best, but the hard part is getting started. Maybe some time . . ."

Once in Italy while wandering through the garden of a villa where I was staying, I stumbled across an ancient sundial which bore this inscription: IT IS LATER THAN YOU THINK.

Those words still return to me when I'm inclined to procrastinate, and I've found it a good idea to recall them on many occasions.

At this very moment it's quite likely ten to twenty pounds later than *you* think.

But it's never too late to do something about it. Just decide when you're going to start.

Today? Tomorrow?

Why put off until tomorrow what you can *take off* today?

What have you got to lose—except those ten, fifteen, twenty, or more pounds?

Aren't you already beginning to see why perhaps the best advice I can give you is, *"Lose Weight—and Live Longer"*?

That you will be more attractive, more glamorous, and more alluring goes without saying.

2

The Stop-Kidding-Yourself
Weight Tables

AFTER CHECKING over the tables, you'll probably feel that the *new* height-weight-frame standards for health and fitness are much tougher to meet than the old, outmoded maximum weight charts.

If you do, you're in excellent company.

So do the FBI agents, whose full-fitness program enables them to slug it out with hoodlums, shoot it out with bank bandits, and stand watch through sleepless nights of surveillance.

The FBI has adopted the findings of this recent study of the Metropolitan Life Insurance Company. Many of the agent force are big, husky, former star athletes. But are they allowed to kid themselves into thinking that an extra-large frame justifies excess poundage?

They are not.

Being overweight is reason enough for a man to be assigned to limited duty—until he gets himself in shape again.

J. Edgar Hoover is now sixty-five years old, and in his

THE STOP-KIDDING-YOURSELF WEIGHT TABLES

Women

HEIGHT (in stocking feet)	SMALL FRAME	MEDIUM FRAME	LARGE FRAME
4 ft. 9 in.	94–101 lbs.	96–110 lbs.	106–122 lbs.
4 10	96–104	101–113	109–124
4 11	99–107	104–116	112–126
5 0	102–110	107–119	115–130
5 1	105–113	110–122	118–133
5 2	108–116	113–126	121–138
5 3	111–119	116–130	125–140
5 4	114–123	120–135	129–145
5 5	118–127	124–139	133–147
5 6	121–131	128–139	137–149
5 7	124–135	132–142	140–153
5 8	128–138	136–146	145–158
5 9	132–142	140–150	147–162
5 10	134–145	144–155	150–165

Men

HEIGHT (in stocking feet)	SMALL FRAME	MEDIUM FRAME	LARGE FRAME
5 ft. 3 in.	118–125 lbs.	124–136 lbs.	132–148 lbs.
5 4	121–129	127–139	135–152
5 5	124–133	130–143	138–156
5 6	128–137	134–147	142–161
5 7	132–141	138–152	147–166
5 8	136–145	142–156	151–170
5 9	140–150	146–160	155–174
5 10	144–154	150–165	159–179
5 11	148–158	154–170	164–184
6 0	152–162	158–175	168–189
6 1	156–167	162–180	173–194
6 2	160–171	167–185	178–199
6 3	164–175	172–190	182–204

NOTE: Adapted from the Metropolitan Life Insurance Company. Derived primarily from data of the Build and Blood Pressure Study, 1959, Society of Actuaries.

thirty-sixth year as director of the FBI. He is nearly six feet tall, and weighs around 169 pounds. A few years ago his weight crept up to over 200, but it didn't stay there very long.

He got busy and lost thirty-one pounds in four months on a diet which cut out bread, butter, and potatoes. In commenting on his own health program, he says, "I have to keep fit. I can't say one thing to the men on the force, and then do the opposite myself, or I'd undermine my reputation."

These new weight standards are applied to special agents on desk duty in Washington as well as to those actively engaged in tracking down criminals.

There are 125 men in the Criminal Investigation Division in Washington. At present all are listed as having desirable weight, according to the "Stop-Kidding-Yourself Weight Tables."

How do *you* rate?

You can find the best and most becoming weight for your height frame according to the very latest Metropolitan Life Insurance tables on p. 17.

I prefer to call them the "Stop-Kidding-Yourself Weight Tables" because it's a pretty safe bet that you *have* been kidding yourself.

3

Why Are You Overweight?

THIS IS A STREAMLINED AGE. Compact cars. Book digests. Shows of the month. Records of the week. Singers of the hour. How do *you* fit into it?

If the song, "June Is Bustin' Out All Over" makes you feel self-conscious and causes you to tug at a too-tight girdle ...

If your clothes often split at the seams, and you blame it on poor workmanship or material ...

If you've gone on countless diets, lost a few pounds, and immediately eaten them back on again ...

If you've resigned yourself to wearing matronly dresses because nothing else fits you ...

If you've decided that no diet ever really works for you ...

And if you think it's simply your fate to be fat ...

Then the following chapters most certainly are for you ... *and you* ... AND YOU!

In fact, this whole book is for all of you women whose grace and loveliness are hidden by folds of unsightly flesh and unnecessary flabbiness, and who long to be lithe and graceful again.

It's also for you men whose waistline has gone to pot, and who have slabs of suet where your muscles should be.

How did you get this way? It wasn't done overnight. It took months and years of careless eating habits, of—let's face it!—eating too much, or at least of eating too much of the wrong kind of food. Fate had nothing whatever to do with it. Neither are your glands to blame, except in a very few exceptional cases.

And heredity isn't the culprit, even though you may claim that overweight runs in your family. Nonsense! Habits of overeating do run in families, but you don't inherit them from your chubby parents or tubby aunts and uncles. Habits, good or bad, are acquired, not inherited, and they can be broken.

It was Thomas Edison who said, "There's one good thing about mistakes—they don't have to be permanent!"

The same is true of habits. They don't have to be permanent. And that extra weight you're carrying around doesn't have to be permanent, either.

You can exchange bad eating habits for good ones, and in doing so, trade obesity for slenderness. You can re-educate your appetite, or, as Dr. Norman Jolliffe termed it, "reset your appestat."

First, though, let's do a little soul searching and find out why you eat too much.

Have you a *fat personality?*

It doesn't sound very attractive, does it? But many psychiatrists have recently gone on record as saying that the overweight person's personality differs greatly from that of the slender person. Contrary to public opinion, the fat man or woman is not a happy one.

There is a close tie between overweight and emotional

stress. "The personality," claim the experts, "produces the fat. Overweight is simply an indication that the personality is maladjusted. Overeating—particularly the overeating of sweets—is often a means of trying to compensate for an unhappy home life, a feeling of inadequacy, or failure in business or love."

The United States Public Health Service decided to look into this subject. An obesity-personality study was held at the Boston Dispensary in the New England Medical Center. Dr. Benjamin Kotkov, a clinical psychologist, was in charge. He was assisted by a psychiatrist, Dr. Stanley S. Kanter, and an internist, Dr. Joseph Rosenthal.

Working with the subjects in groups of six at a time and employing psychology's best methods of testing personality, including the Rorschach ink-blot test, the doctors arrived at these conclusions:

1. The fat subjects had poorly adjusted personalities. They were more introverted and less friendly than the slender subjects. They were less able to utilize their energies to win friendship, success, or love.

2. The overweights spent more time daydreaming and less in action than the normal weights, and they tended to be nervous, anxious, and neurotic.

3. Their own intense self-absorption made them insensitive to the reactions of others. When they became annoyed they turned their anger inward, which resulted in moodiness and depression.

4. If they lost in friendship or love to someone else, they were more grief-stricken and desolate than a normal-weight person would be. They crept into a shell and brooded over real or imagined wrongs, instead of working them off or fighting them out.

5. Tense and miserable, unsure of themselves, the fat group did not enjoy social relations as much as others did,

nor did they make any effort to promote new friendships.

"Their fear of failure is too great," Dr. Kotkov says. "Their basic personality problems must be solved and confidence in themselves attained. Otherwise they will go on eating for consolation and will refuse to stick to a diet."

As much as you hate to do it, you might as well admit that you're overweight because you consume more calories in food and drink each day than you expend in energy. Now, ask yourself this question: *"Why do I overeat?"*

Dr. Charles S. Freed, another authority on obesity, has one answer. He says, "Most overweight persons use eating as an emotional outlet. Anything that increases their emotional tension (such as sorrow, anxiety, nervousness, or irritability) increases their desire for food."

What is *your* particular problem? What are the frustrations that make you turn to food for compensation? Is it insecurity, unhappiness, a feeling of inadequacy, boredom, or rejection?

What are you running away from?

Whatever it is, here's some good advice from Dr. George Lawton, author of *Aging Successfully:* "Look at it this way—if you were drinking too much or resorting to drugs, you'd probably realize that you were seeking escape from reality. *Overeating is the very same thing . . . Get rid of the terrible necessity to find in food your major satisfaction in life.* (Italics mine.) Your first *new* interest can be a search for something that will really interest you."

"But I *do* have a new interest now," you may say. "I'm really interested in losing weight. I've let myself go for so long that I'm anxious to lose it in a hurry."

Perhaps you look around for a crash diet. You don't have very far to look. Newspapers, magazines, and books are full of them.

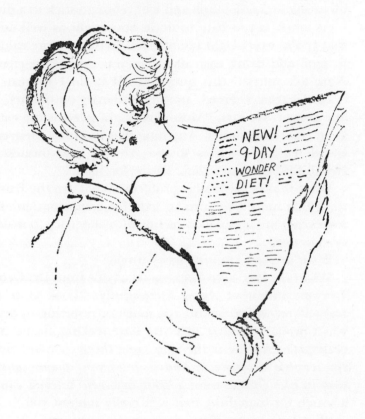

NEW!
9-DAY
WONDER
DIET!

Enthusiastic fat friends are eager to share with you the secrets of their latest miracle diets.

"My dear, this one's absolutely marvelous," they will tell you. "You just eat rice three times a day and think yourself thin. You can take off five pounds in five days, ten pounds in ten days, there's no limit to it. It's like a game."

It's like a game, all right. A game of put-and-take in reverse. You take off a few pounds and you put them right back on again.

Why is it that these friends with sure-fire crash diets are still fat?

I'll tell you why.

They starve themselves for a week and lose weight, but they become so ravenous on a poorly balanced diet that they eat up everything in sight the following week.

And they do it virtuously, smugly, saying, "After all, I lost five pounds last week—I can pamper myself a little bit."

So they pamper themselves right back into the lost five pounds, plus three or four more.

I don't believe in miracle diets.

And don't *you* believe that you can just sit back and think yourself thin, either. The success of your diet may very well depend on the way you condition your mind to it, but it takes a positive mental attitude combined with action to get results. Or, as somebody wiser than I once expressed it, *"Faith—with work."*

Find out your particular reason for overeating and start working on it. Is it monotony? Then look for new and different ways to do your work. Even the dullest task may hold a challenge if you search for it.

If you're a housewife, leave the dishes in the sink, take the children, and go on an impromptu picnic once in a while. Fresh air and sunshine are good blues-chasers as well as beauty-builders.

Perhaps you feel that your family and friends don't appreciate you. Maybe they don't. Find out the reason for it, and try showing *them* so much affection and understanding that they'll have to respond. Stop feeling sorry for yourself and start realizing your tremendous potential as a real personality—and I don't mean a *fat personality*.

Disraeli, the famous English statesman, said, "Nurture your mind with great thoughts, for you will never go any higher than you think."

I'd like to paraphrase that remark to read, "Nurture your mind with beautiful thoughts, for you will never be any more beautiful than you think." Nor any thinner, either!

A negative attitude and the fear of failure can hold you back, slow you down, or stop you completely.

They can make you say, "Oh, what's the use?" and reach for the hot biscuits and gravy and chocolate cream pie.

But a positive approach will help you to hold that mental picture of the slender, vital person you want to be—the person you can be!

Start this very moment by visualizing the way you want to look and mentally seeing yourself achieving that goal. Outline your purpose in writing, work toward it, and never give up or let the thought of failure enter your mind.

How much do you want to lose? Five pounds—or fifty?

Whichever it is, keep this thought in mind: There is one *sure* way of getting slim—and *staying* slim—not for just a month, not for just a year . . . but for a lifetime!

4

Don't Be Calorie-Wise
and Pound-Foolish

YOU HAVE a pretty fair idea of what calories are, and of what too many of them do to you. You'd like to cut down on them, avoid them, or boycott them completely.

You cannot build a picket fence around yourself and hang a sign on it saying, *"Calories, Keep Out. This Means You!"* It wouldn't do any good if you could.

You meet them constantly at breakfast, luncheon, dinner, and cocktail parties. Calories are the unseen guests at every meal you eat, at each nibble that you sneak with a fine disregard for them.

This includes a growing number of people—growing in numbers as well as avoirdupois!—who have a quaint theory, "What nobody sees me eat won't make me fat."

But a calorie isn't fooled by such shenanigans. So since you can't lick 'em, join 'em. Make friends with them, recognize their temperamental differences, and let them work *for* you instead of against you.

Let's be specific for a moment, in a simple, nontechnical sort of way.

A calorie is the measure of the energy value of food—and also of your body's energy requirements.

If you eat more calories than you burn up by work, worry, play, or exercise, where can those extra, unwanted calories go?

Where, indeed, except to be stored as fat, located in various and unbecoming places?

What are your own personal daily calorie requirements? That depends on several things.

You need from 14 to 20 calories per pound of body weight, *based on what your normal weight should be.*

By just lazing around the house you burn up about 14 calories per pound of normal body weight. Delightful, isn't it?

Nature also lets you use up a fair amount of calories during the night while you do nothing but sleep, breathe —and maybe snore.

But wake up and smell the coffee. Drink it black with no sugar, and let's get back to reality.

If your work involves light exercise, you use up 16 calories per pound. And if your activities are strenuous— which is doubtful—you'll burn 18 to 20 calories per pound.

Let's assume that you're an average person whose work consists of light exercise which burns up 16 calories per pound.

Multiply your normal weight by 16. Wait a minute—I said your normal weight, which means what you *should* weigh—not your present weight. That excess fat on your otherwise lovely frame is lazy, inactive tissue. It does no work and burns no calories, so include it *out.*

Let's say that your normal weight should be 130 pounds, but you actually weigh 160 and want to lose 30 pounds of it.

Figure on the basis of the weight you want to be. Multiply 130 by 16. It comes to a nice even figure, 2,080. This is your daily maintenance number of calories.

"But I don't want to *maintain* my weight," you say. "I want to *lose* it!"

Of course you do. And you will lose, safely, steadily, and surely.

Most balanced reducing diets range from 1,000 to 1,500 calories a day. An in-between figure, 1,200, is a pretty good average.

You're allowed 2,080 calories a day just to keep your present weight. I know—I heard you. And I haven't forgotten. You want to shuck off thirty pounds and be slim and sylphlike again.

And you can be. All you have to do is to cut your allowed number of calories down by 500 to 1,000 per day and you'll lose between one and two pounds a week.

To stay as plump as you are, how many calories are you allowed? That's right—2,080. So what happens if you go on the 1,200-calorie diet?

You don't need a Univac machine to figure it for you. Subtract 1,200 calories from 2,080 and you get 880. That's 880 calories of stored fat that you'll use up each day you're on the diet, or 6,160 calories a week.

Since it takes about 4,000 calories to make a pound of body fat, on the 1,200-calorie diet you'd lose one and a half to two pounds a week, more or less, depending on your fluid balance (water retention) and other factors which we'll discuss later.

On the 800-, 900-, or 1,000-calorie diet you'd naturally lose faster. But if you're past thirty and need to lose more than ten pounds, you'll look younger and feel better if you keep to a steady loss averaging no more than two pounds a week.

If you're a housewife, you may say, "Look, I work hard

all day long, cooking, cleaning, washing dishes, ironing—
surely I can allow myself more than the sixteen calories
per pound of my weight!"

I hate to have to tell you this, but here are the facts:

1. Housework is classified as *light* exercise.

2. Housework uses the small muscles of the body (those
of the hands, arms, feet, and legs), and in his book, *Food
and Health,* Professor Henry C. Sherman says, "Moderate
use of large muscles may easily involve a larger expenditure
of energy than does the most intense use of a set of much
smaller muscles."

3. You think ironing is hard work and should use up
at least a few thousand calories? Sorry to disillusion you.
Ironing takes a mere .87 calories per pound of body weight.
If you weigh 130 pounds, you'd have to iron for an hour
to burn up the number of calories you'd consume in a
medium serving of applesauce.

If you're a man, maybe you've decided that you want to
get rid of the excess weight brought on by our push-
button age.

"From now on," you say, "whenever I can I'm going to
walk instead of ride, and climb the stairs instead of taking
an elevator. That'll take all this extra weight off me!"

It's a good idea if it works. It's still a good idea if it
won't work. And it won't.

Do you know how many steps there are from the first
floor of the Empire State Building to the 103rd floor? I
didn't know either until I looked it up.

I'd thought of counting them personally, but changed
my mind when I found out that it meant trudging up
2,240 steps.

That's a sizable jaunt for any fellow with the fortitude
to try it, and you'd expect to lose five or six pounds in
such a climb, wouldn't you?

Well, you wouldn't. From the time you started the climb until you collapsed on the 103rd floor you would burn no more than 2,000 calories, resulting in a skimpy weight loss of one half pound.

It isn't worth the effort, is it? I'm not selling exercise short. It's an excellent conditioner, but it isn't the answer to weight reduction.

Calories alone are the key to successful reducing. *Cut your daily calorie intake by one third and you will lose weight.*

But wait a minute before you start slashing calories indiscriminately. Don't be calorie-wise and pound-foolish. Spend your calories wisely and outwit the pounds.

You know that the fuel foods are fats, carbohydrates (sugars and starches), and proteins (meats, fish, poultry, cheese, eggs, and all dairy products).

But here's the catch in spending your calories: one ounce of fat contains two and one fourth times as many calories as one ounce of the other two food elements.

An ounce of fat packs a weighty 255 calories. An ounce of protein or carbohydrate contains only 113 calories.

It's easy to see why fats must be restricted on a diet. But carbohydrates have to be dealt with cautiously, too. Recent experiments have shown that persons who put on weight easily have a defective mechanism in their bodies *for handling carbohydrates.*

All starches and sugars have to be broken down into glucose by your digestive juices before they can be used by the body. If your body fails to supply the substance needed to convert carbohydrates into energy they will be stored as unused fat.

But here is the fat boy's bonanza, the chubby girl's blissful bonus: If you eat an ounce of protein instead of an ounce of carbohydrate, although each has 113 calories, a small miracle takes place. *Protein's specific dynamic action steps up your metabolism and enables you to burn up to 130 to 140 calories!*

A high-protein diet will whip up your metabolism so that combustion of fat for energy increases—and you lose weight faster.

By eating meat, eggs, fish, poultry, low-fat cheese, or yogurt three times a day you keep your metabolism going in high gear, prevent a drop in blood sugar which often causes a craving for sweets, and avoid hunger pangs which lead to overeating.

According to Dr. Roger J. Williams, University of Texas biochemist and president of the American Chemical Society, there is a vital area of the brain which is apparently an automatic appetite control mechanism. It's called the hypothalamus.

You didn't know you had one?

It is a built-in contraption which, when it's happy and well-behaved, keeps you from overeating and getting as big as a hippopotamus.

And do you know what makes a happy hypothalamus?

I'll tell you. It's protein. The little fellow hankers for protein for breakfast, lunch, and dinner. If you eat at least one of the complete protein foods at each meal you'll keep this handy appetite control in shape to control *anything,* even the most ravenous appetite.

On a high-protein diet you'll lose weight faster, have more vitality, and retain a firm skin and excellent muscle tone as you reduce. And you won't have that empty, all-gone-in-the-middle feeling. Protein does away with those gnawing, do-or-diet hunger pangs that you get on fad diets.

Unlike fat, protein can't be stored in the body, yet you must have it each day of your life to repair and renew worn-out cells and tissues. *Protein is the only substance which can do this.*

Perhaps some day a bright young chemist will come up with a formula for a protein food supplement which will be as successful as the vitamin and mineral supplements we now have. But that time is still in the future, along with trips to the moon. *Protein is obtainable only in the food that you eat.*

A high-protein diet protects your health as it causes a weight loss of deposited fat and water, which is what you want to lose.

But if you go on a protein-deficient diet you will lose weight at the expense of vital tissues. You will invite premature aging, loss of health and attractiveness—and perhaps endanger your very life.

Your protein intake should be between 80 to 100 grams a day at any time, and this is especially important on a reducing diet. Four hundred calories of the complete protein foods will give you approximately 100 grams.

You needn't worry about getting the right amount of the other two food elements, since an excess of either of them is stored as fat.

Trim each sliver of fat from your lamb chops or steak, and be sure that they're broiled instead of fried. Eggs should be poached, boiled, or scrambled in a double boiler, with no butter or other fat.

Fresh fruits and vegetables can supply all the natural sugars and starches your body needs.

Here are some proved, effective, calorie-wise ways to outwit the pounds:

1. *Eat protein three times a day.* And that means breakfast, too, even though you're a confirmed breakfast-skipper. Meat or eggs for breakfast will step up your metabolism so you'll burn more calories than you consume. Your blood

sugar will remain on an even level and prevent the hunger pangs that cause you to grab a sweet roll or doughnuts in midmorning, or overeat at luncheon.

2. *Restrict fats.* That includes butter, cream, whole milk, gravy, sauces, and salad dressings. Let your use of fats (which should be limited) include vegetable fats rather than animal. Safflower oil is the very best type of fat which should be directly consumed, as it balances out the hidden fats eaten in meat and aids in preventing the possibility of fat accumulation. A small amount of safflower oil may be mixed with lemon juice or vinegar and used for a salad dressing.

3. *Cut down on carbohydrates.* I'm tempted to say, "Cut out carbohydrates," since almost all fatties overeat them. Eat fresh fruits and vegetables as natural sources of sugars and starches, but use discretion in choosing them. Eat liberally of the low-carbohydrate fruits and vegetables, moderately of those containing medium amounts, and sparingly of the high carbohydrates. (The carbohydrate content of fruits and vegetables is listed in the next chapter.) *Foods containing white flour and white sugar are taboo.*

4. *Eat plenty of the bulky, low-calorie fruits and leafy vegetables.* They include cabbage, spinach, letuce, endive, escarole, cauliflower, broccoli, sauerkraut, asparagus, celery, tomatoes, apricots, oranges, grapefruit, and melons. These fill up the empty spaces, provide roughage to combat constipation, and are good sources of important vitamins and minerals.

You don't have to starve yourself to wage an all-out war on overweight.

The only safe and sure way to get slim—and *stay* slim— is to learn which calories are your friends and which are

your foes. Learn which calories will work for you, and
which will loaf on the job and allow fat to accumulate.

Then write it on your mental memo pad—
Engrave it on your calorie-wise consciousness—
"Protein calories are a fatty's best friend!"

5

The Fattening Fifteen

THERE'S A WORD for the good-for-nothing man who is too lazy to work and doesn't do enough to earn his keep.

He's a bum.

There are calorie bums, too.

They are good-for-nothing calories that never do an honest day's work and contribute nothing whatever to society or the individual—except fat.

Nutritionists call them "empty calories." They're the calories that fatten you up while they starve you to death.

The foods which contain them may be pleasant to taste and beguiling in appearance, but don't be fooled by them. They fail to provide your body with the nutrients which are absolutely necessary to sustain life.

These calorie bums are potential killers.

When you fill yourself up with the empty calories of candy, cake, pie, pastry, sirupy soft drinks, and alcoholic beverages, you destroy your appetite for the health-giving protein-, vitamin-, and mineral-rich foods.

You become overweight and undernourished.

White flour, white sugar, and fats are refugees from a

calorie chain gang. These particular bums are partners in crime with that recognized Public Enemy and Killer-at-Large, overweight.

They are the nutritionists' nightmare—and the girdle manufacturers' delight.

Overweight is like a purse-snatcher at night. It overtakes you when you're not looking. It's something that you believe happens to other people, but not to *you*. You can see that your friends are gaining weight, a little bit here and a little more there. But you, yourself? Certainly not! The scales are a liar and the laundry shrinks your clothes.

It takes a little while before you concede that *all* the scales can't be in cahoots against you. You decide not to sue the company that put the preshrunk label on your garments.

Finally you say, "Everybody I know is on some kind of diet. Why should I be different? That 1,200-calories-a-day deal seems OK to me. Looks like there's plenty to eat on it, so I won't have any trouble sticking to it."

You shouldn't have. It's a balanced diet and there's certainly no reason for you not to stay on it. You won't go hungry and you will lose weight.

But watch out!

If you're careless, forgetful, or cheat on purpose, you can easily run your 1,200 calories up to 2,000 before you know what's happening. What about that butter you doused on your vegetables? Just from force of habit, wasn't it?

And you've always used cream and sugar in your coffee, so surely just a little won't hurt. Only a teaspoonful of sugar and a tablespoonful of cream in each cup of coffee. And how many cups of coffee do you drink a day? Five or six? More?

You're supposed to eat fruit as often as possible for

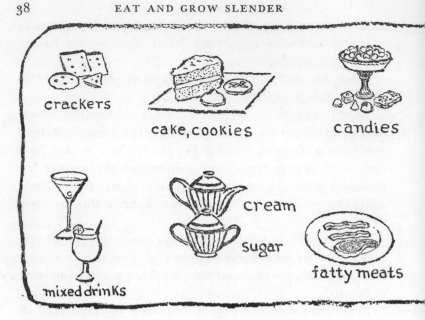

crackers

cake, cookies

candies

cream

sugar

mixed drinks

fatty meats

dessert, and you're out of fresh fruit. But there's a can of peaches on the shelf. So you open them up and eat them, heavy sirup and all. You could have washed the sirup off, you know. Never thought of that, did you?

And don't forget the tablespoonful of jelly you had for breakfast, and the French dressing on your luncheon salad.

"Why, that's no food at all," you say.

It certainly isn't, nutritionally speaking.

But these calorie bums can boost your intake by several hundred calories and sabotage your diet completely.

If you really want to lose weight, look better, and live longer, here is a list of foods to avoid.

How many of them do you eat, and how often? Seldom, frequently, or every day?

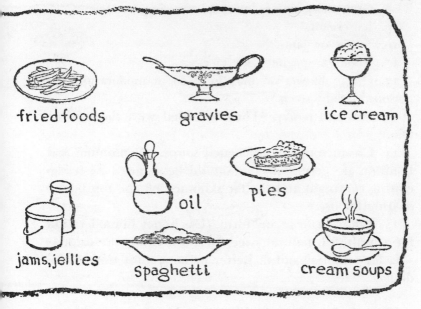

fried foods   gravies   ice cream

oil   pies

jams, jellies   spaghetti   cream soups

The Fattening Fifteen

1. Bread or crackers.

2. Cake or cookies (or other products made with a combination of that terrible trio, white flour, white sugar, and shortening fats).

3. Candy or chocolate in any form.

4. Cocktails. (Look out for their high calorie count, especially in the sweet ones.)

5. Cream. (That includes custards and puddings made with cream and sugar. Junket made with powdered skim milk is all right.)

6. Fatty meats. (And trim off the visible fat from all meats.)

7. Fried foods.

8. Gravy, rich sauces, or salad dressing.

9. Ice cream.

10. Jellies or jams.

11. Noodles, spaghetti, or rice.

12. Oil. (Safflower oil may be used in moderation, for reasons already given.)

13. Pies and pastry. (They're loaded with the terrible trio.)

14. Cream soups or thickened soups. (Consommé and bouillon are permitted, but should be defatted by refrigerating overnight and the fat skimmed off the top before heating for use.)

15. White sugar in any form. (Use honey in moderation for a healthful, natural sweetener, but count the calories —62 for a tablespoonful. Better make a scant teaspoonful do.)

"Everybody's always telling me what *not* to eat," you say, "and you've summed the whole thing up for me. Now, what I want to know is this—what *can* I eat?"

Plenty.

And you won't have to follow the advice given by comedian Jack E. Leonard, either. After he had lost about a hundred pounds he told his friends the secret of his diet.

"Eat all you want," he said. "Just don't swallow it!"

Here are some of the foods that you can eat—and swallow—while you lose weight.

Almost any lean meat, except pork which should be avoided. If your purse permits, you may have broiled steaks, lamb chops, roast beef, or roast lamb every day.

But a high-protein diet needn't be expensive. Equally good are broiled hamburger and baked meat loaf (fortify both with skim milk powder for extra protein and flavor) or cubed steak simmered in fat-free bouillon, which can be made by dissolving a bouillon cube in a small amount of water.

The organ meats, such as broiled liver, baked heart, broiled kidney, or sweetbreads, should be eaten twice a week.

Tired of meat? Then have roast or broiled chicken, baked, broiled, or poached fish, cottage cheese or yogurt served in a variety of ways with either fruits or vegetables, and eggs, soft-cooked, hard-cooked, poached in skim milk or tomato juice, or scrambled in a double boiler with a little skim milk but no butter.

What else? Fresh and frozen vegetables and fruits, naturally. Have them raw in salads or cooked—but never overcooked—in a small amount of water, with no butter and very little salt.

No, salt isn't high-caloried itself, but it retains up to 70 times its weight in water. One teaspoonful of salt used in cooking or sprinkled on your food holds 70 teaspoonfuls of water in your tissues.

So cut down on salt. Unless you want to stay fat and water-logged.

These vegetables are recommended for a reducing diet:

Group I (3 per cent carbohydrate)

Asparagus	Lettuce
Beet greens	Mushrooms
Broccoli	Mustard greens
Cabbage	Radishes
Cauliflower	Spinach
Celery	Squash, summer
Chicory	Swiss chard
Chinese cabbage	Tomatoes
Cucumber	Water cress
Endive	Zucchini
Escarole	

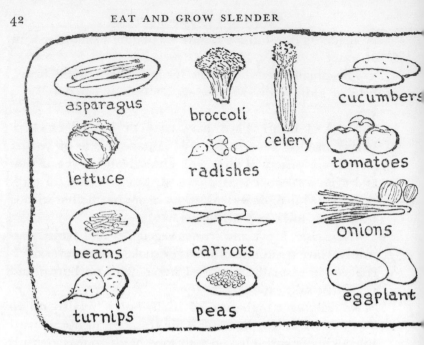

Some Foods You Can Eat

Group II (no more than 9 per cent carbohydrate)

Artichokes	Kohlrabi
Beans, green	Lamb's-quarters
Beans, wax	Okra
Beets	Onions
Brussels sprouts	Peas, fresh
Carrots	Peppers
Collards	Pumpkin
Dandelion greens	Rutabagas
Eggplant	Squash, winter
Kale	Turnips

Some of the following fruits which may be included in your diet contain more than 9 per cent carbohydrate, but

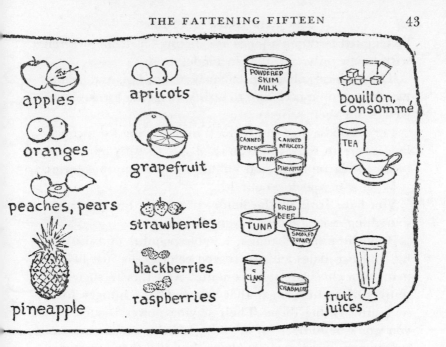

apples | apricots | POWDERED SKIM MILK | bouillon, consommé
oranges | grapefruit | CANNED PEACH | CANNED APRICOTS | PEAR | PINEAPPLE | TEA
peaches, pears | strawberries | TUNA | DRIED BEEF | SMOKED TURKEY
pineapple | blackberries | raspberries | CLAMS | CRABMEAT | fruit juices

they are *natural* sources of starch and sugar at a compara-
tively low calorie count:

Apples	Peaches
Apricots	Pears
Blackberries	Pineapple
Cherries	Plums
Currants	Raspberries
Grapefruit	Rhubarb
Loganberries	Strawberries
Melons	Tangerines
Oranges	

Cranberries, gooseberries, lemons, and limes are allowed, but I hesitate to list them only because you may

be tempted to dump a lot of sweetening on them. Sweeten with honey only, and that in moderation.

The high-carbohydrate bananas, dates, figs, and raisins may be eaten on occasion, to satisfy a craving for sweets as well as for their satiety value.

Let's suppose that you feel a frantic craving for a chocolate ice-cream soda, and you're all set to dash out to the nearest soda fountain and gobble up 400 empty calories.

What can you do about it?

You have fruit in the house, of course, but you want something sweet, and you want it *now*.

A medium-sized banana, a tablespoonful of raisins, a fig, and two dates add up to 200 calories, or just half as many as a chocolate soda contains. And they're such rich sources of natural sugar that you won't be hungry for a soda after eating them. Their staying power is such that you won't be hungry for anything else for some time.

Don't go overboard on them, but use them to stop a craving for sweets and chisel a calorie—or 200 calories—whenever it's necessary.

"All right," you say, "I can quit using extra salt and butter. Your high-protein diet gives me plenty of meat, fish, poultry, low-fat cheese, vegetables, salads, and fruits. I think I can cut out the fattening fifteen—with one exception. Do you *have* to include cocktails in the list? What are you, a teetotaler?"

No, I'm neither a teetotaler nor a tippler. If a highball before dinner or a glass of dry wine with your meals can be included in your calorie count for the day, go right ahead and have it. Just don't let it take the place of your *protein* calories. But don't kid yourself into thinking that liquor won't make you fat.

I'm reluctant to give the calorie count of cocktails because they vary greatly, depending on the bartender's generosity and the measurements used.

Here's an *average* estimate of highballs made with a one and one-half ounce jigger of liquor and plain soda or water (add 100 calories if you use ginger ale):

Scotch	108	calories
Bourbon	135	"
Rye	118	"
Brandy	112	"

And a rough estimate of popular cocktails:

Daiquiri	124	calories
Dry Martini	143	"
Eggnog (1 punch cup)	338	"
Flips	250	"
Manhattan	167	"
Old Fashioned	183	"
Planter's Punch	177	"
Rum Sour	163	"
Tom Collins	182	"

That's enough for you to see that the mixed drinks are not for you if you have a weight problem.

A glass of dry wine can be managed on a low-calorie diet. Claret, Burgundy, and sauterne have about 75 calories in a three and one-half ounce glass. The same amount of the sweet wines (port, sherry, and Tokay) contains about 130 calories.

Look at it this way: a Manhattan cocktail normally contains 167 calories, which is bad enough. But a heavy-handed host can easily run it up to 200 calories. If you drink three of these potent ones, half your day's calories are shot.

And you're feeling half shot.

So you get reckless or forgetful or both, and dive with abandon into the tray of canapés.

Oops! That does it. Before you can say, *"pâté de foie gras* on toast," or "anchovies, olives, and bacon," *two* day's worth of calories go down the gullet.

What one small boy learned in school could serve as a lesson for you. He came home and told his parents, "I learned about liquid measurements today. Four gills make a pint, two pints make a quart—"

"And then what?" his mother asked.

"Then I asked the teacher, 'Where does the jigger come in?' " he said. "And you know something? The jigger doesn't come in at all!"

That's the way it should be if you really want to lose weight. Cocktails remain on the fattening fifteen list.

And the jigger doesn't come in at all.

6

How To Diet If You Have No Will Power

You rule your family with a whim of iron. Kindly, but firmly, in a no-nonsense sort of way.

You're adamant in business deals.

In the midst of world-shaking crises you make adamant look like whipped cream.

Come hell, high water, or hysterics, you're still the master of your fate, the captain of your soul.

Except—

When you're confronted with hot, homemade rolls slathered with butter and fresh preserves . . .

Or faced with a plate heaped temptingly with devil's food cake and ice cream . . .

Or surrounded by cream pies, French pastries, and bowls of chocolates and bonbons . . .

Then what happens?

Does your whim of iron remain in good working order?

Is your will power still holding out in the face of temptation?

It's like handing a starving man a bag of popcorn and saying, "Now, eat just *one* grain."

The odds are overwhelmingly against your being able to control yourself.

What can you do about it? There are several ways and means. Find the one that works successfully for you and stick to it, or figure out a combination of them to use as the occasion demands.

Eliminate. This is the Spartan method of simply cutting out the forbidden foods. If you can do it you don't need will power. You have enough "won't power" to get you by. It's a fine, noble technique which is worth trying part of the time. But if you're more human than noble you'll find this rough going for the long haul.

Substitute. For each of the fattening fifteen that has to go, find a satisfactory substitute. This takes imagination and ingenuity, as well as some family co-operation, but it can be done. It's the best way to diet if you have no will power—or even if you have. The substitution method satisfies your appetite and helps to retrain it at the same time. I recommend it highly.

Sublimate. You can't eat everything in sight and get slim—or stay slim. Next to eating, what's your favorite recreation? Develop it. Concentrate on it. Cultivate some new hobbies. Get absorbed in doing something that really interests you, and your mind won't tick off the minutes until the afternoon chocolate malt break or the next meal. You don't have to spend a lot of money to cultivate a hobby. It can be something simple, such as bird-watching.

Or girl-watching (if you're a man).

Recapture the eagerness of childhood and relive the times when you were having so much fun that you forgot to eat. Never let boredom make you overeat.

If somebody tells you, "Oh, go fly a kite!" do it. It might be fun.

Pinpoint your particular food weakness. You probably know what it is, even if you haven't admitted it. Bring it out into the open and face it. Is it bread that you can't resist? Perhaps it's dessert. Anything and everything sweet, the sweeter the better. Or is it butter, cream, gravy, rich sauces, and salad dressing?

Decide what your forbidden food downfall is, and plan what to do about it—avoid it, substitute for it, meet it head-on with no holds barred, or outsmart it.

Stock a low-calorie shelf. This method combines substitution and elimination. Throw out those boxes of cookies, cake mix, and pudding. Toss away the sugar bowl and the jars of jam and jelly. If they're left around the house, sooner or later you're going to eat them.

Accept the fact that you haven't any will power where food is concerned, and get rid of the items that tempt you.

You can fill all that nice empty space on your shelf—and in your stomach—with low-calorie substitutes. Here are some suggestions:

Honey for sweetening. It takes such a little bit to satisfy that the calorie content needn't be high, but don't overdo it on any concentrated sweet. Honey contains important minerals, some of the B vitamins, and enzymes that aid digestion. It's also an excellent energizer.

Powdered skim milk. What did dieters ever do without it? It supplies your diet with all of the protein, vitamins, and minerals that whole milk does (with the exception of vitamin A) at half the calorie cost. You won't have to give up whipped cream, if you'll make it with powdered skim milk. Directions are given on the boxes or jars of the various brands, whether they're called powdered skim milk or nonfat dry milk. If you can't drink black coffee or tea, try using one or two teaspoonfuls of powdered skim milk. Better dissolve the milk in a small amount of cool water first, or it may lump in the hot liquid. You'll get extra protein, calcium, B vitamins—and a good taste. Use powdered skim milk for cooking, drinking, to make low-calorie fresh fruit milk shakes, and in a multitude of ways which will be mentioned from time to time.

Bouillon cubes, instant bouillon, and instant consommé. A cup of hot, low-calorie soup will take the edge off your appetite and help prevent overeating. Calorie cost is very low on these—from 2 to 9 calories a cup. It is good for the midafternoon slump, too.

Assorted teas, including Chinese, Russian, and herb teas. Who says you can't have a variety of drinks with no calories at all? If you want to fancy them up and sweeten them (with a spoonful of honey), you can still stay within your calorie budget. Serve with some of these for extra flavor: a slice of lemon stuck with cloves, a slice of orange and a dusting of cinnamon (or a piece of cinnamon bark if you can get it), crushed fresh mint leaves, two or three small pineapple chunks, a few fresh strawberries or raspberries, or fresh or canned (without sugar) black cherries. Any of these add a luxurious touch and a fine flavor to an otherwise calorie-free drink.

Canned fruits, water-packed or juice-packed, with no sugar. Fresh fruit is better for you, with frozen fruit a runner-up, but for your emergency shelf you might stock these canned varieties: applesauce, apricots, blueberries, boysenberries, cherries, fruit cocktail, grapefruit, oranges, pears, peaches, pineapple, raspberries, and tangerines.

Hungry for a different dessert, simple but satisfying, and low in calories? Combine small mandarin orange sections with black cherries and raspberries, then top with gingered whipped cream (made with powdered skim milk) and a sprinkle of toasted coconut.

Or take a plain dish of applesauce, surround it with two

or three apricot halves and pineapple fingers, pour over it a sauce made with orange juice and honey, and dash a bit of nutmeg on it. Easy—and delicious.

Canned protein. The fresh foods are always preferable, but canned items are quick, convenient, and good to have on hand to satisfy a sudden hunger when you're out of fresh food, or if you have unexpected guests and no time to get to the market.

Albacore, bonito, chicken, crabmeat, clams, dried beef, lobster, shrimp, tuna, salmon, and turkey are all high-protein, low-calorie foods. But remember to buy diet-pack tuna and salmon, or else wash off the oil before serving.

Are you a Dagwood sandwich addict? You won't have to give them up if you'll make them like this: two thin slices of Provolone cheese, one slice of chicken or turkey, one slice of dried beef, and a middle layer of lettuce and tomato.

Where's the bread?

You mean that dry stuff that sticks in your throat for a moment—and on your hips for a lifetime?

There isn't any. And you won't even miss it. The Provolone cheese provides the top and bottom layer of this streamlined Dagwood sandwich, protein-packed and filling.

Or have a roll instead of a sandwich. Take your choice of sandwich filling—meat, chicken, turkey, fish, or cheese —spread it on a lettuce or cabbage leaf, roll up, and fasten with a toothpick.

You see? You *can* have sandwiches and rolls without bread.

Fruit and vegetable juices. Eat whole fruit whenever possible, but keep the following on hand to make revitalizing vitamin cocktails or fruit and skim milk shakes:

apricot nectar, clam, grapefruit, grapefruit-orange, orange, pineapple, pineapple-grapefruit, sauerkraut, tomato, and vegetable blends. Read the labels to see that no sugar is in them.

A later chapter will give recipes for liquid meals.

Miscellaneous. Have on hand assorted herbs, assorted spices, gelatin (plain), cider and herb vinegars, bottled lemon juice, lime juice, garlic and onion juice, low-sodium salt, horseradish, mustard, and soy sauce.

For your refrigerator shelf. Reserve space for safflower oil, cottage cheese, and yogurt in an assortment of flavors.

Safflower oil is the only fat that you should allow yourself on your diet. It's a good source of lecithin, vitamin E, and linoleic acid which are necessary for life itself.

It also helps prevent water retention in your tissues, and speeds up your weight loss by causing your body to change sugar to fat more slowly.

It lessens your craving for sweets and prevents hunger pangs by causing food to remain in your stomach longer. Use one or two tablespoonfuls a day mixed with lemon juice or cider vinegar, and whatever seasoning you like, for a salad dressing.

There's a much publicized cottage cheese "blitz diet" which is reported to cause a weight loss of three to five pounds in two days. Breakfast, lunch, and dinner are the same for both days: 1 cup (8 ounces) of cottage cheese with 3 peach halves. Or you may substitute 1 small orange, 7 apricot halves, ¾ cup of fresh berries, or 1 small cantaloupe.

If you prefer vegetables instead of fruit, you may have cottage cheese garnished with green pepper, onion, radishes, cucumber, tomato, or water cress.

But if you have no will power and couldn't eat the same thing at each meal for two days, have it for one meal a day. Cottage cheese is high in protein, calcium, and other nutrients, with most of the fat removed. An 8-ounce serving, which is a man-sized, filling amount, contains 230 calories. And don't forget that protein calories whip up your metabolism so you burn up more calories than you consume!

Yogurt, like cottage cheese, is another almost perfect food. It builds up your body—yet aids in banishing fat. High in protein, low in butterfat, easily digested, it kills harmful bacteria in the intestines and promotes the growth of health-giving, *friendly* bacteria. It was known even in Biblical times, and today it is perhaps one of the world's greatest health foods.

Dr. Elie Metchnikoff, Nobel prize winner and head of the Pasteur Institute in Paris, was the first to do extensive research on yogurt, and introduced its health-giving qualities to Western Europe.

Princess Alexandra Kropotkin, well known in this country as an author and for her interest in diet, credits yogurt with saving her life when she was a little girl. Exiled from Russia and living in England, she became desperately ill with a summer dysentery. It was yogurt culture, sent from Bulgaria in liquid form and added to milk, which cured her and made her the enthusiastic yogurt booster that she is today.

Use yogurt as a substitute for sour cream and save a third on calories. Add a bit of mustard and horseradish to it as a sauce for meat, or chop crisp cucumber and onion in it to serve with fish. Combine it with chili sauce for a Thousand Island dressing.

Eat yogurt plain or with any kind of fruit or raw vegetable salad. For an excellent regulator, make a prune whip yogurt for your dinner dessert, or have it for a bedtime snack. If you're famished for a sweet dessert, chop a few dates in vanilla yogurt and drizzle a little honey over it.

You already know that dates, figs, and bananas are high-carbohydrate fruits. But because of their natural sugar content and high satiety value a small amount satisfies, and they are permitted in moderation.

For an exotic dessert, try fresh mangoes or papayas, if you can get them, topped with orange yogurt sprinkled lightly with ginger. If these tropical fruits aren't available, substitute fresh persimmons. And if *they* aren't in season, combine fresh or canned greengage plums and seedless grapes with the same topping.

Only a lack of imagination can limit the art of substitution. Browse through a health food store and make some discoveries of your own. You may find cookies which contain no flour, fat, or sugar, and candies made of fruits, honey, and sunflower or sesame seeds. If you like chocolate, look for carob powder (also called St. John's bread), which is a fine and healthful chocolate substitute. Do your own exploring and become acquainted with the numerous foods that are low in calories, but high in nutrition and taste appeal.

Dr. David B. Hand, speaking at a convention of nutritionists, warned them, "Don't take the fun out of eating. A diet that's a grim business won't work."

The dull, no-fun diet is difficult for *anybody* to stay on. If you haven't any will power it will be impossible for you. To get slim and stay slim, avoid monotonous meals. Make eating a gay, festive occasion. And whenever possible, add dash to your diet with at least one new, imaginative, low-calorie but luxurious type of food.

7

The Educated Nibble and
the Slimming Snack

HAVE YOU A tubby hubby in your home? Or a chubby child?

You have? Then, as a wife and mother, what are you doing about it?

"Why should I do anything?" you ask. "What if my husband and child are pleasingly plump? We're happy the way we are. Besides, my husband is still a little boy at heart—he's just never outgrown his baby fat!"

Then it's high time he did.

Listen to what one unhappy overweight person said recently in an interview for a national magazine: "I was a child and a teen-ager with 'baby fat' and a large appetite. Now I'm thirty and still have the 'baby fat.' I believe it is just a matter of habit—*an early overeating habit. But my mother could have helped me.* Instead she worked at ignoring the problem. I can't urge parents strongly enough *to help their children now.*"

Life for the fat boy or girl can be a friendless, frustrated existence. They are unable to compete with other children in sports and games. They lack the competitive spirit, the ambition and energy that mark the leaders of their class. They are slow in action, generally slow and timid in expressing their thoughts, and often the victims of inferiority complexes and emotional disorders.

And on the physical side, Dr. James M. Strang, of the University of Pittsburgh's School of Medicine, warns, "Heavy bodies wear down weak legs and feet. Cardiac disorders are aggravated. There are also disorders such as hypertension and diabetes."

A ten-year survey made by the federal and state departments of agriculture and public health reveals this frightening fact: One child out of every four in America is dangerously overweight.

One child out of every four whose health is endangered by obesity. Shocking, isn't it?

Doctors agree that something must be done about it. But what?

The responsibility rests almost completely on you mothers.

Dr. Alfred George, in his book, *Your Weight and Your Life,* says, "Obesity in an adult can often be traced to infancy or childhood. A common pattern can be traced to a family setting that characteristically exaggerates the emotional significance of eating . . . It is the mother who becomes the dominating influence in the emotional life of the children. She tries to realize in them the dreams of luxury and idleness of which she felt deprived in her own childhood. In a symbolic way, she is making up to herself for those deprivations *by overfeeding her children.*" (Italics mine.)

"I *want* my husband and children to eat well," you say. "It's part of my job to see that they're well cared for and well fed, isn't it?"

Indeed it is. And it's a very gratifying job, too.

But let's get one thing straight: what do you mean by "well fed"?

Do you mean giving them all that they can eat of balanced, nutritious meals which include the protein of meat, fish, poultry, eggs, low-fat cheese, and certain other dairy products, as well as the vitamin- and mineral-rich fruits and vegetables?

Or . . . do you mean stuffing them to bursting with high-starch macaroni, spaghetti, noodles, white rice; the fat-laden gravies, thick soups, cream sauces; and the so-called "reward foods" of childhood, such as candy, cake, cookies, pastries, and ice cream?

Stop and take stock of your family's food habits. If they are undesirable ones, it's up to you to change them.

You've already learned about the fattening fifteen. What are you going to do about them—eliminate, substitute, or sublimate?

You'll have to work out your own solution. You might eliminate the worst offenders, substitute for the others, and ferret out various family projects that will create interest, discussion, or even cheerful dissension.

With a rousing, friendly argument or game going on nobody will sit brooding over Mom's hot biscuits and gravy, or drool in dreamy anticipation of whipped-cream pie for dessert.

Never urge second helpings on a family of fatties. And before they have a chance to ask for more, have the last course of fruit, cheese, or melon ready to set before them.

What about in-between-meal snacks? Have them, by all means. They're a fine idea. And they're fun.

"What are you saying?" you ask. "You just told me never to serve second helpings to a fat family. And now you say, 'Oh, sure, snack between meals!' You're rather inconsistent, aren't you?"

Not at all.

The slimming snack can help you and your overweight husband and children to lose weight.

Just be sure that the between-meal nibble in your house is an *educated* nibble. That means the nibble or snack that's satisfying enough to relieve hunger pangs, prevent overeating at mealtime, and supply low-calorie nutrients as well.

The educated nibble contains no calorie bums. Its calorie content is a hard-working crew which stokes your metabolic furnace, aids in burning up fat, keeps your blood sugar on an even keel, and provides needed energy. It can be a small piece of low-fat cheese, a thin slice of cold meat, chicken, or turkey, a hard-cooked egg, three or four tablespoonfuls of cottage cheese or yogurt, or a glass or skim milk or buttermilk.

If you have after-school icebox raiders or midnight snackers in your home, make it easy for them to find slimming snacks. Fix a tray of crisp carrot sticks, celery, radishes, cucumber, raw cauliflower, or whatever raw vegetables you have on hand—even raw turnips are delicious. Keep fresh fruit in the front of the icebox, and chilled cans of unsweetened fruit juices to drink plain or mix into milk shakes—made with low-fat powdered skim milk, of course.

If your chubby child is absolutely famished for a chocolate malt, try this: add three tablespoonfuls of carob powder to a glass of buttermilk, mix in enough yogurt to thicken, then whip it up in a blender until it's smooth and creamy. (For other healthful drinks see Chapter 11.)

Here's how to make a protein-, vitamin-, and mineral-rich banana split that's substantial enough for a full luncheon. Blend together to a fluffy, creamy mixture one-half cup of cottage cheese with three ounces of fresh skim milk. Slice a banana lengthwise and put two scoops of the chilled, creamy cheese on it. Top one mound with fresh sliced peaches (if they're not in season crushed pineapple is good) and the other with crushed fresh or frozen strawberries or raspberries sweetened with a little honey.

"What about appetite depressors?" you ask.

Don't waste your money. There's a well-known candy appetite depressor on the market which is presumably a low-calorie, vitamin-fortified sweet. It's a caramel type of candy and each piece contains about 30 calories, which isn't particularly low. The diet candies are expensive and have little to recommend them. You still have to cut your calories to lose weight, with or without any of the aids or depressors, so why bother with them?

"But I've found that something sweet between meals takes the edge off my family's appetite," you say, "so that they're satisfied with less food."

You're quite right. It does.

In diet experiments at the Brusch Medical Center at Cambridge, Massachusetts, it was proved that taking sugar before meals depresses the appetite. Most mothers already know this and for years have cautioned their offspring, "Don't eat candy before dinner—it'll spoil your appetite!"

But when an appetite *needs* spoiling it's a different story.

"In proper amounts," Dr. Charles Brusch says, "sugar seems to quiet the body's craving for food."

So have something sweet for a slimming snack and an appetite depressor. But have it in the form of *natural* sugar.

For the adult, a cup of herb tea with a spoonful of honey is satisfying and energizing. And for both adults and children, one or two high-carbohydrate dates or figs, or a few grapes with their natural sugar content, serve the same purpose.

The beloved Kate Smith was a chubby child. Irregular hours and poor eating habits during her long radio career increased her weight problem.

"I ate when I had an opportunity," she said recently. "Frequently I sent out of the studio for food. I'd order thick chocolate malts, ice cream, cookies, cakes, and chocolate bars."

Years of this type of snacking finally caught up with her, and her doctor's ultimatum frightened her into action. "Lose weight and get your blood pressure down," he said, "or I'll no longer take the responsibility for your health."

She went on a diet of 1,000 calories a day and at the time of this writing has taken off 85 pounds. Within the next year she is determined to lose 40 pounds more, or a *total of 125 pounds.*

Since slimming down she has more energy and looks more attractive than ever before in her professional life.

"Each day is like a gift of gold," she says. "I'm lucky to be alive. But don't expect me to tell you how much I weighed before starting to diet. Even though I'm a big girl—nearly six feet tall—I'm embarrassed to admit my former weight."

Her doctor reminded her that she'd gone on diets before and never stayed on them. He doubted whether she'd last on another one, and it was his doubt that spurred her on.

"It was just the challenge I needed," she says. "There was no great mystery about taking off my excess weight. It was simply a matter of limiting my intake to 1,000 calories a day. I found I was able to do this without going hungry."

For breakfast she usually eats a poached egg, some kind of fresh fruit, a piece of toasted whole wheat or gluten bread, and tea or caffeine-free coffee.

"I often have cottage cheese for lunch," she says, "or a fruit salad or leafy green salad, with a glass of skim milk or buttermilk. At dinner I have green vegetables and lean meat—lamb, beef, or fowl. No duck, goose, or pork—too much fat."

Even on a calorie intake of 1,000 a day she has enough left over for a slimming snack of tomato juice or skim milk before going to bed.

"My blood pressure had to be lowered or I was headed for a stroke," she says. "By going on a diet, changing my way of life to a more relaxed, leisurely pace and learning moderation in all things, I lost weight, regained my health, and now feel better than I have in years."

Dr. Charles Glen King, executive director of the Nutrition Foundation, has this warning for overweights: "Seven out of ten leading causes of death and crippling disease are associated with the condition of being obese."

Dr. King blames a lack of nutritional knowledge and the misleading "hard sell" of the advertising business for much of America's overweight. Devitalized, overprocessed foods and pastries made with white flour, white sugar, and lard are prettily packaged to tempt the gullible customer. No manufacturer or advertiser is going to put a label on these foods which says, *Not Fit for Human Consumption.*

Of course they aren't, but nobody will tell you so.

And lose all that beautiful business? I should say not! It's up to you, as a homemaker, to develop sales resistance. To shape your meals—and reshape your fat family—around the complete proteins of meat, poultry, fish, eggs, low-fat cheese; the slimming snacks of raw vegetables; low-calorie beverages (never the sirupy, carbonated drinks!). And, of course, fresh fruits, which contain all the *natural* sugar you need.

Show your family the advantage of eating today for a brighter *and lighter* tomorrow.

Whether our nation is undermanned and underarmed is for the experts to decide. But perhaps our deadliest danger lies in the fact that we're overweight and over-stuffed.

Man invented the wheel, conquered the wilderness, blazed trails through the skies, chained the lightning and made it speak—but has himself become a slave to those man-made tools, the knife and fork.

As newspaper columnist Inez Robb says, "We may be in deadly peril from the intercontinental ballistic missile, but it is my honest opinion that the French fried potato will destroy us first . . .

"Let's get the starch out of the stomach and return it to the backbone where it belongs."

8

How To Burn Up Body Fat

IF YOU EAT two slices of bread a day over and above your energy requirements, you will gain from fifteen to twenty pounds a year, depending on your size and metabolic rate.

Just 100 to 150 extra unneeded calories a day, and in twelve months' time you wonder where your figure went.

Nutritionists, doctors, insurance companies, and, unfortunately, coroners, have proved that the longer your belt line the shorter your life line.

To hold a short belt line and a long life line you must maintain a balance between your food intake and your energy output.

But you don't eat bread at all? Fine! Just don't forget to count that extra pat of butter on your vegetables, the second and third cup of coffee with cream and sugar, or the dollops of gravy and mayonnaise.

Any of these can add up to 50 calories or more. And 50 extra calories a day which aren't used up for energy can add seven pounds to your weight in a year.

"Seven pounds in a year?" you say. "Why, that's nothing to worry about—and please pass the butter!"

Maybe it isn't—at least not at the moment. But keep it up for seven years and by that time you'll be a whopping fifty pounds heavier. Give or take a pound or so. Not to mention being fifty pounds less attractive, less energetic, less healthy, and less happy.

The fallacy still persists that fat people are happy—chubby, cheerful cutups who think that it's fun to be fat.

Then why are more than thirty million Americans either on a diet, starting a diet, or planning to start one tomorrow?

Here is a United Press news story from Gibsonton, Florida, which tells the sad story of one fat person who always seemed jolly, headlined, CIRCUS FAT LADY ENDS HER LIFE. "Circus fat lady, Dotty Blackhall, 52, famed for her sideshow appearances with Ringling Brothers' Barnum & Bailey Circus, is dead. Police said that Mrs. Blackhall, who reportedly weighed 500 pounds, apparently took her own life because of ill health."

"Maybe it was her age," you say. "Maybe she felt that she was getting older and didn't have much to look forward to."

Maybe. But age certainly had nothing to do with the despondency felt by a group of Canadian teen-agers recently. Education Minister Dunlop of Ontario rejected the admission of eight girls and two boys to Long Branch Teacher's College in Oakville because they were overweight. "A person who is overweight is not in good health," he said, "and the education department wants only teachers who are." One of the students who was dismissed for reasons of health was a boy of nineteen who weighed 278 pounds. Mr. Dunlop added that he had written a personal letter to each of the students rejected from the college, and I fervently hope that he suggested a weight-reducing program designed to improve their health and their chances for the future.

I'd like to add my own personal plea to these disappointed youngsters and to all of you with weight problems in any age group:

"Stop overeating and start living!"

By the time you've reached the age of twenty-five, your body requires about 1 per cent less food each year to maintain its basal metabolic processes such as heart action, breathing, digesting, and the business of living.

Metabolism is your body's chemical process that transforms what you eat into energy.

As you grow older your body slows down and requires less food. Unless you reduce the amount of food that you eat, increase your physical activity, or step up your metabolism, the result is an inevitable gain in weight.

"I don't understand why I'm getting fat," you say. "I eat exactly the same way I always have—no more and no less."

That's precisely the trouble. The same amount of food that kept you slim at twenty can make you plump at thirty and fat at forty.

If your metabolism has slowed down and you fail to convert to energy the calories you consume, they are stored as fat.

There aren't any calorie piggy banks where you can save the surplus calories you eat for leaner days. I wish there were. You can save them all right, but they'll be stored in fat depots on your thickening body, and there won't be any leaner days for you.

If you saw wood, chop down trees, or dig ditches, you may use up 4,000 calories a day compared to an office worker's 2,500 or the average housewife's 2,200.

Dr. Herbert Pollack, chairman of the nutrition committee of the American Heart Association, gives this explanation of the weighty problem to women: "Not too long ago the housewife spent 240 calories scrubbing the family wash and another 50 calories hauling it to the line. Today, dumping the clothes in the automatic washer and tapping a button takes no more than 50 calories."

Today's housewife, with her various labor-saving appliances, is probably expending nearly 1,000 fewer calories a day than her mother and grandmother did.

Dr. Pollack doesn't mention the modern male's chores, but it's a pretty safe bet that wood sawing, tree chopping, or ditch digging aren't included in his daily activities.

It isn't the single day's calorie binge that's disastrous. *The thing to watch is your lifetime eating pattern.*

Learn the law of energy intake-output, and realize that when you steadily eat more calories than you expend in energy you're storing up body fat which, unlike money, is easy to save but hard to spend.

The rate at which you burn energy—your basal metabolism rate—may be either high, low, or normal. If it's low you will tend to put on weight easily.

The worrier uses up more energy than the placid person. Haven't you noticed that the slow-moving, easygoing person is usually plump and the tense, nervous one is thin? Worry takes more energy than brain work does. Nervous tension is produced by worrying, hurrying, fussing, fretting, and under a severe strain the energy output may be increased 10 to 20 per cent. The calm person moves slowly and deliberately. The nervous person uses up to three times more energy with his fast movements.

At every decade of life your basal metabolism rate decreases and your tendency to put on weight increases. Time and nature seem to conspire to keep us from staying

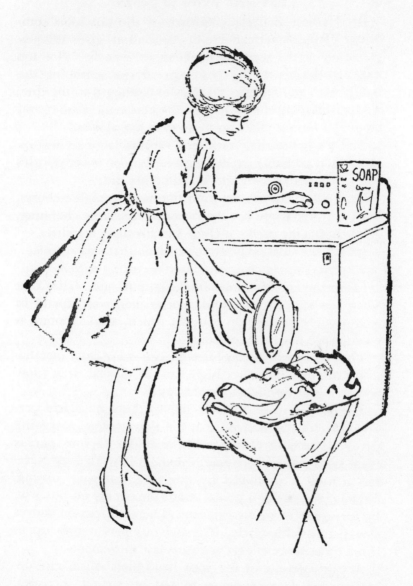

slim and youthful. But sometimes nature manages to compensate for her cruelty. She's provided us with certain
fruits and vegetables that stir a reaction in the body which
aids in burning fat.

"Find out about them," she seems to say. "They are
secret weapons that I've given you to fight fat—use them
to defeat me if you can!"

These fat-fighting fruits and vegetables supply the vitamins and minerals which you must have to form the enzymes needed to burn up body fat and release energy.

When you go on a one-sided diet which features a combination of no more than two or three foods, the important fat-burning enzymes can't be formed.

Here's nature in a kindly mood again: she allows us to
use up some of the calories consumed in food by the mere
process of digesting and assimilating it for the body's use.
The energy cost to the body varies in digesting different
foods.

It costs your body about 25 calories of energy to digest
a cup of cooked celery or two stalks of raw celery. Now,
let's do a little simple arithmetic. That amount of celery
eaten supplies 10 calories—so you burn up 15 more calories on the deal than you take in. The law of intake-output, remember? And you're the winner, by a 15-calorie
margin.

Isn't that delightful? You could eat all day long at that
rate and lose weight in the bargain.

But wait a minute! You must have a well-balanced diet,
so you can't live on celery alone. That's just one example
of the low-caloried vegetables that can help you burn up
fat.

Now let's take a look at the other extreme. Sugar and
alcohol are loaded with calories, *yet the metabolic cost of
digesting them is almost nothing.* They must remain

where they belong—among the list of the fattening fifteen foods to avoid.

Here are some of the fruits and vegetables that will help you burn up body fat:

Apples	Crab apples	Onions
Apricots	Cranberries	Oranges
Artichokes	Cucumbers	Papaya
Asparagus	Currants	Parsley
Beans, green	Dandelion	Parsnips
Beans, wax	greens	Peaches
Beet greens	Eggplant	Pears
Beets	Endive	Peppers, green
Blackberries	Figs	Pineapple
Blueberries	Grapefruit	Plums, damson
Broccoli	Grapes	Pomegranate
Brussels sprouts	Honeydew melon	Quince
Cabbage	Huckleberries	Radishes
Cabbage, Chinese	Kohlrabi	Raspberries
Cabbage, red	Kumquats	Rutabagas
Cantaloupe	Leeks	Spinach
Carrots	Lemons	Squash, summer
Carrot tops	Lettuce	Strawberries
Cauliflower	Limes	Swiss chard
Celery	Loganberries	Tangerines
Cherries	Mangoes	Tomatoes
Chervil	Mushrooms	Turnips
Chicory	Mustard greens	Water cress
Chives	Nectarines	Watermelon
Collards	Okra	

Many of these vegetables are so low in calories that the metabolic process of digesting them uses up more calories than one serving of them contains. Fruits, with a few exceptions such as strawberries, cranberries, currants, and melons, are not extremely low in calories, but they are rich in the vitamins and minerals that form the fat-fighting enzymes.

Chapter 9 will contain a number of vegetables listed in two groups. Those in group 1 will supply you with no more than $12\frac{1}{2}$ calories for each half-cup serving. Even on a strict diet you're allowed to eat these to your heart's content. (Well, almost!)

You know that protein calories are a fatty's best friend, but have you made that knowledge work for you?

Here again are the facts that are important enough to bear repeating. An ounce of fat contains 225 calories. An ounce of protein or carbohydrate each contains 113 calories.

But what a difference the protein calories make to *you!*

Protein's specific dynamic action increases your metabolism so that you burn up to 130 to 140 calories for each 113 that you eat.

Even if you have to take off your shoes to count to 20 you can figure that you'll lose weight at that rate.

Physicians at Bellevue Hospital in New York who have been treating overweight patients believe that it's time for a thorough search into the metabolic approach to reducing.

The Bellevue patients were put on a diet of 1,100 calories a day, but as the study continued, amazing differences in individual weight loss became apparent.

The patients with normal metabolism lost weight steadily and surely. In sharp contrast, only 15 per cent of those with below normal metabolism lost weight. A few maintained the same weight even on a diet, and 60 per cent of the group with low metabolism gained weight.

Your thyroid gland controls your metabolism, which includes your body's use of food and energy. It is your body's thermostat and speed-controller. It slows down or speeds up the rate at which you burn food for energy.

"You were talking about protein," you say. "How does protein affect my body's speed-controller?"

An authority on glands, Dr. Herman H. Rubin, author of *Glands, Sex, and Personality,* tells us that there is a direct linkage of protein with glandular efficiency. He goes on to say that many important hormones and innumerable enzymes, such as those involved in digestion, could not exist without protein.

In the case *for* protein—and *against* carbohydrate—he says, *"Too much carbohydrate overburdens the glands . . . and makes us more liable to overweight and diabetes."*

Protein is the one food that we can't live without. Protein can take the place of the other food elements. It can be converted into carbohydrate by the body, and it can be burned for energy instead of fat. *Yet neither fats nor carbohydrates can substitute for protein.*

Nearly a hundred years ago in London a short, fat man, sixty-six years of age, learned the value of a high-protein diet in reducing. His name was William Banting, and he might almost have been the original Mr. Five-by-Five. He weighed 202 pounds and was only 5 feet 5 inches tall.

He tried to lose weight by every known method of that time. This included diets, Turkish baths, spa treatments, purgatives which left him weak, and violent exercise which made him hungry. He kept right on gaining.

Finally, because he thought he was going deaf, he went to Dr. William Harvey, an ear, nose, and throat specialist. This doctor, far ahead of his time, put Banting on a completely new type of diet. Within several months on his new diet Banting lost nearly fifty pounds, and reduced his waist by more than twelve inches. He was able to tie his own shoelaces again. The balloonlike paunch which kept him from seeing his feet and forced him to inch downstairs backward had disappeared.

He was a new man—and the new man was delighted.

He wanted to share his miraculous diet, which shed weight and renewed vitality, with everybody who needed it.

In 1864 he published a small book, *Letter on Corpulence,* addressed to the public and containing his diet. Here it is:

> Breakfast: Four or five ounces of beef, mutton, kidneys, broiled fish, or cold meat of any kind except pork. One small biscuit or one ounce of dry toast. A large cup of tea without milk or sugar.
>
> Lunch: Five or six ounces of any fish, any meat except pork, any vegetable except potato. Any kind of poultry or game. One ounce of dry toast. Fruit. Dry wine, such as claret or sauterne, was permitted.
>
> Tea: Two or three ounces of fruit. A piece of rusk. A cup of tea without milk or sugar.
>
> Supper: Three or four ounces of meat or fish, as for lunch. Dry wine, as desired.

William Banting had plenty to eat on his diet. It was not especially low in calories. *But they were mostly the protein calories of meat, fish, and poultry, with no carbohydrate except for the amount contained in his small portion of dry toast or rusk, and the natural sugar and starch in fruits and vegetables.*

The basic rules of his high-protein diet, with some modifications and additions, can be as effective for you as it was for this ex-fatty of the nineteenth century.

At the risk of being called a spoilsport, I would advise limiting the dry wine to one glass a day, and adding a glass or two of buttermilk, nonfat milk, or a half cup of yogurt or cottage cheese. These would supply needed calcium, which was lacking in Banting's diet.

Heat and sunlight can aid in burning up body fat. A hot tub bath of ten to fifteen minutes can raise your temperature as much as 2 degrees. Body fuel is burned up by whatever means that produces body heat, and some of that fuel which you burn will be fat.

You expend more calories in digesting a whole orange than you do in drinking the juice.

A brisk walk or mild exercise, particularly before breakfast, will whip up your metabolism. You haven't the energy for it? Nonsense! Such a routine will *give* you energy. Save your slimming exercises for a more convenient time, but do a few stretches, bends, and twists, and feel yourself come alive as you take the kinks out of lazy muscles.

An air bath, advocated long ago by Benjamin Franklin, is a good metabolism-waker. Get some air and sunlight on your bare body, even if you have to lie on the floor to keep out of sight of peeping Toms.

Let's review once more the importance of protein in your diet:

1. Protein's specific dynamic action stokes the body fire (increases metabolism) and burns up fat deposits.

2. Without protein the body is unable to make certain hormones and enzymes which involve energy exchange reactions.

3. Worn-out tissue cannot be repaired and wounds will fail to heal if the body is not provided with sufficient protein.

4. The skin, hair, nails, vital body chemicals, a considerable part of the blood, and all organs and soft tissues are made principally of protein. Only by eating the complete proteins of meat, fish, poultry, eggs, low-fat cheese,

skim milk, and yogurt can they be kept in good condition.

5. Protein at each meal (and the occasional educated nibble) will keep the blood sugar level high and prevent the almost uncontrollable hunger which leads to overeating and overweight.

6. Immediately after eating your metabolic fires burn brightly, gradually going down as the time between meals lengthens. Keep those fires burning steadily—and burning up fat!—by eating three high-protein, low-fat, and low-carbohydrate meals a day. You'll lose weight faster this way than if you skipped meals or put yourself on a semi-starvation diet. *Don't skip meals when dieting or at any other time.*

And you'll look younger, feel better, and have more vitality as you slim down in this sensible, safe, and *permanent* way.

The Take-Your-Choice Diet

You're the independent type. You like to make your own decisions and you hate to be told exactly what to do. You'll take suggestions, but if anybody tells you precisely what you must or must not eat for each meal you get a chip on your shoulder.

"Who does this guy think he is?" you ask. "Telling me that I have to eat this on Monday, that on Tuesday, and whatever he says all the other days of the week. Doesn't he know that it isn't always convenient or practical to stick to a rigid diet?"

Indeed I do know. That's why I believe that the best long-range results come from having a flexible eating plan. A basic pattern that allows you to eat everything that you want, *except* . . .

Remember the fattening fifteen foods?

If you've forgotten, go back to Chapter 5 and reread them. Better still, write them on a card to carry with you. Let that card be your reminder, your diet counselor— and your conscience.

76

Eat what you like, within moderation, except for those forbidden foods.

When you're dining out, tell the waiter not to serve bread and butter before the meal. If you have to nibble, order celery and radishes, or have your salad brought first, California-style. Skip the thick, creamy soups and have tomato juice, fruit cup, or crab or shrimp cocktail. You don't need to eat all of the sauce, but there's good, fat-fighting protein in the crab and shrimp.

If you *must* have a cocktail, why not order Compari (pronounced kom-*pah*-ree) and soda in a tall glass with a twist of lemon? Compari is a sweet Italian vermouth which costs you only 50 calories.

White Dubonnet with soda is another refreshing calorie-saver. If you want to save both calories and money, try Rhine wine (or sauterne or Riesling) and seltzer for a champagne substitute. A glass of dry wine isn't a bad choice, but a tall drink lasts longer and seems more festive.

Let's suppose that you're dining at Chasen's in Beverly Hills, California, surrounded by beautiful and slender motion-picture and television stars. Joan Crawford might be sitting next to you eating one of the broiled steaks which gave Chasen's its fine reputation. (Steak and tomatoes three times a day are Joan's favorite reducing foods.) But you'd do well to consider the delicious and unusual fish on the menu—prawns, Dover sole, English turbot— or any of the many other delectable and low-caloried foods from the sea.

If you prefer to go to Romanoff's, another star-studded restaurant, you'll be greeted by Prince Mike himself. And he's seen to it that the menus will please his friends, the diet-conscious stars. Romanoff's curried crab, cold sliced tenderloin, and spinach salad are especially popular with weight-watchers.

Dessert is wheeled in by cart, and you have a choice of *pots de crème* (for those who don't *care* what shape they're in) or a variety of fresh fruit for you ... and *you* ... and *me*.

You see how it is? Wherever you go you can use your Take-Your-Choice Diet.

Nobody's going to twist your arm and *make* you eat roast goose or beef Stroganoff when you're dining out. You can always get broiled or roasted meat or chicken and baked or broiled fish. You can even have a hamburger sandwich—minus the mayonnaise and bun, of course— or a hot dog without the trimmings, but with tomato, mustard, or relish to zip it up.

If you crave the gourmet touch and feel absolutely famished for beef Stroganoff you can make it at home. Follow the standard recipe. But instead of the sour cream sauce, substitute a low-calorie version. Make it this easy way:

Blend 1 cup of yogurt with ½ cup of hot consommé. (Use more consommé if you want a thinner sauce.) Pour over the beef and let simmer until thoroughly heated.

This amount makes enough sauce for four delicious servings. Add a little horseradish or mustard for extra flavor. Here's a protein-enriched accompaniment for many meats—much better than ordinary sauces or gravies (which you shouldn't have anyway!)

You need never go hungry or thirsty on the Take-Your-Choice Diet.

For a midmorning or afternoon refresher with no calories at all you may have hot or iced tea or coffee, or plain soda with a lemon twist or a dash of lime. Hot bouillon, hot consommé, or either one on the rocks with a slice of lemon have so few calories that you don't have to count them.

For a protein pickup and for a sleep-inducing nightcap with less than a hundred calories, try a glass of buttermilk, skim milk, or half a cup of yogurt. A variety of protein pickups and vitamin cocktails are given in Chapter 11.

You may eat absolutely all you want of these:

Raw Vegetables for Salads
or the Slimming Snack

Cabbage	Escarole
Cauliflower	Lettuce
Carrots	Pepper, green
Celery	Radishes
Chicory	Romaine
Cress, garden	Tomatoes
Cucumber	Water cress
Endive	

A balanced diet which supplies you with sufficient protein, vitamins, and minerals to safeguard your health, yet remains within your calorie limits, is essential. The yellow and leafy green vegetables are good sources of vitamin A, and you need a minimum of two servings a day. By choosing your vegetables from the low-calorie groups listed below, you can have half-cup portions of four vegetables from Group 1 *and* two from Group 2 for an *average* of 100 calories—or the same number of calories you'd consume in one potato or one-half cup of lima beans.

You take your choice—but it's up to you to choose wisely!

Group 1

Extremely Low Calorie Count

Asparagus (6 stalks)	Collards
Bean sprouts	Dandelion greens
Beans, string	Mushrooms
Beet greens	Mustard greens
Broccoli	Poke greens
Cabbage	Rhubarb
Cabbage, Chinese	Sauerkraut
Cauliflower	Spinach
Celery	Squash, summer
Chard	Turnip greens

Group 2

Very Low Calorie Count

Bamboo shoots	Leeks
Beets	Okra
Brussels sprouts	Rutabagas
Carrots	Scallions (6 small)
Eggplant	Tomatoes, fresh or canned
Fennel	Tomato juice
Kohlrabi	Turnips

Fruits, with a few exceptions, average 50 or more calories a serving. But they are rich in the vitamins and minerals which form the fat-fighting enzymes, and must be given a high place on any diet. Oranges, grapefruit, and strawberries are rich in vitamin C which can't be stored in the body and must be supplied daily. You need a minimum of one citrus fruit and two other fruits a day.

Here are the most desirable fruits and size portions for the weight-watcher:

Fresh Fruits

	CALORIES (approximate)		CALORIES (approximate)
Apple (small)	50	Pear (medium)	50
Banana (½ medium)	50	Pineapple	
Blackberries (½ cup)	30	(½ cup, diced)	35
Blueberries (½ cup)	40	Plums (2 medium)	20
Cantaloupe (½ med.)	50	Orange (small)	50
Grapefruit (½ small)	50	Orange juice (4 oz.)	60
Grapefruit juice (4 oz.)	45	Raspberries (½ cup)	35
Honeydew melon		Strawberries (1 cup)	45
(2-inch slice)	50	Watermelon	
Muskmelon (½ med.)	50	(small slice)	100
Peach (medium)	50		

Frozen fruit, unless sweetened or packed in sirup, has the same calorie count as fresh fruit. Watermelon, usually considered low in calories, actually contains 25 calories per standard one-half cup. Better serve one-half to one cup, scooped out as melon balls, or it can sabotage your diet. The large wedge which is generally served will cost you 250 calories.

Canned, Water-Pack Fruits

	CALORIES		CALORIES
Applesauce (½ cup)	50	Peaches (2 halves)	50
Apricots (½ cup)	35	Pears (2 halves)	50
Cherries (½ cup)	40	Pineapple (1 slice)	35
Grapefruit sections		Plums (3)	30
(½ cup)	35	Raspberries (½ cup)	50

Plan your meals by taking your choice from the basic foods needed for health, youthfulness, and vitality.

1. Have at least one of the complete proteins at each meal. These include lean meats (with the exception of pork), the organ meats—liver, kidneys, and sweetbreads—fish, poultry (except duck or goose, which are too fat), eggs, and dairy products, especially the low-caloried buttermilk, skim milk, cottage cheese, and yogurt.

2. Vegetables, either raw or cooked. At least one serving each of the leafy green or yellow vegetables, and more as desired from Group 1.

3. Fruit. Preferably fresh, but frozen or water-pack may be substituted when necessary. At least one citrus fruit daily for vitamin C. Take your choice of two others.

4. Green salads. Two teaspoons of safflower oil may be mixed with lemon juice or apple cider vinegar for a dressing, with seasoning or herbs to taste.

5. Honey for sweetening, when necessary. But count the calories—65 for a tablespoonful—and don't overdo it.

6. Bread. Only if you *absolutely must*. Not more than two thin slices daily, with whipped cottage cheese instead of butter for a spread. Take your choice of the whole-grain varieties, or for fewer calories, Jerusalem artichoke rusk, or the rye hardtack type such as Ry-Krisp or Norwegian flat bread.

Is the Take-Your-Choice Diet safe for overweight teenagers?

A sixteen-year-old girl, Kathryn Shallcross of Wynnewood, Pennsylvania, answers the question in her own words.

"Last year I was a teen-age hippo weighing 240 pounds," she says. "I was really ashamed. But I dieted and lost 100 pounds in less than six months. I'd like other young girls to see that it can be done!"

When Kathryn weighed 240 pounds her diet was high

in fats and carbohydrates. She ate four or five slices of buttered toast, coffeecake, or rolls and butter with each meal. She put away huge amounts of fried eggs, bacon, and peanut butter and jelly sandwiches. She thought nothing of drinking eight or nine glasses of milk or as many cups of cocoa a day. Her after-school refreshments were malted milks, pies, cakes, and ice cream. Dinner was whatever her mother served, with second helpings of everything, including dessert. And of course there was always a TV or bedtime snack—a few more sandwiches and a slice or two of cake or pie.

Then a boy came along, and he didn't like fat girls. Kathryn was so far off the road to Sylphsville that she had to do something. The fattening fifteen had to go. She began to take her choice of all the nonfattening foods, and to apply the power of positive shrinking. It wasn't easy the first few weeks, but she had an incentive. She chose to be slim and attractive instead of fat and lonely.

Here are the Take-Your-Choice meals that Kathryn ate while she was shedding one hundred pounds:

BREAKFAST

   Choice of: 1 orange, ½ grapefruit, **or orange juice**
   1 small glass of milk
   1 egg, boiled or poached
   1 slice diet toast, lightly buttered

LUNCH

   Choice of: hamburger on ½ roll, or cottage cheese and
      tomato salad, or 2 hard-cooked eggs
   1 glass milk
   Fresh fruit

DINNER

Any lean meat, broiled or roasted
Large portions of any low-caloried vegetable
Lettuce and tomato salad (no dressing)
Choice of: ½ grapefruit, or simple custard, or junket, or
gelatin

AFTER-SCHOOL AND TV SNACKS

Choice of: celery and raw carrots (any raw vegetable
from the low-calorie list would be all right), or fresh
fruit

Never, never skip breakfast on any diet.

One of the complete proteins of egg, meat, or cheese
should start your day. A protein breakfast will keep your
blood sugar on an even level and your metabolism stepped
up. It will provide energy and prevent a midmorning
letdown, hunger pangs, overeating at lunch, low morale,
jitters, general crankiness, and other breakfast-skipper's
complaints.

If you've never taken a good vitamin and mineral food
supplement, now is an excellent time to start. My personal choice is a formula called Nutri-Time. You may wish
to look into it for your use.

Hal Boyle, newspaper columnist, lost forty pounds in
ninety days without feeling starved, without losing his
strength or sense of humor, and without feeling sorry for
himself. He did it by cutting out the fattening fifteen and
by fortifying himself with two vitamin supplements a day.

His doctor told him, "Take a couple of vitamin pills a
day. Cut your liquor to two highballs a day, but don't
take any medicines. You don't need them."

"Well, doc," Hal said, "two drinks a day is taking
medicine—for it sure ain't drinking."

He went on the wagon altogether and cut out all sweet desserts.

"No cake, pie, or ice cream," Hal said. "I even quit chewing bubble gum with my daughter."

He limited himself to one piece of rye or whole-wheat bread a day. If he ate a sandwich for lunch he went without bread the next day.

"I cut my usual portions in half," he says, "and took my choice of lean meats (all fat cut off), eggs, cottage cheese, and filled up on plenty of raw and cooked green and yellow vegetables. They told me that if I slimmed down I'd have the girls at the office standing in line. I do, too. But all they whisper in my ear is, 'What's your secret, Skinny? I'd like to lose a little weight myself.' "

Let's go back to an early Stoic philosopher for an answer. "All philosophy in two words," said Epictetus, "sustain and abstain."

Sustain your health, strength, and vitality with your choice of high-protein and vitamin-and-mineral-rich foods (with added supplements, for good measure).

And abstain from the fattening fifteen.

10

The Count-Your-Calories Diets

CRASH DIETS are not on my list of effective reducers.

The extremely low-caloried meals shortchange you on needed protein, vitamins, and minerals unless every precaution is made in planning them.

You may lose five pounds in one week, but you gain them back the next. Unless you stabilize your diet according to your energy output, this off-again on-again practice can continue indefinitely. You keep right on losing the same five pounds and gaining them back over and over again.

You don't have to be told that this isn't the way to get slim and stay slim.

Or do you?

Maybe you just need to be reminded occasionally. Instead of starting out with the lowest number of calories consistent with health and energy, let's reverse the usual order of diets.

Let's begin with 1,400 calories a day.

86

Unless you're below average in height and very inactive, you should be able to lose a pound or more a week on 1,400 calories.

"But what if I don't?" you ask. "What good will it do if I can't lose weight on it?"

You'll have set your appestat lower, as Dr. Norman Jolliffe expressed it. You'll have curbed your unruly appetite gradually and painlessly for the next drop in calories, which will be less difficult for you because of this.

Now, if necessary, you're ready for the 1,200-calorie diet, or whatever suits your own particular requirements. If you're small and inactive or have an unusually low metabolism, it may be that 1,000 calories a day will work best for you.

Fluid balance (water retention), metabolism, and body chemistry vary greatly with each individual. Exaggerated claims are made for some quickie diets—"Lose five pounds in five days, or ten pounds in ten days!" They don't bother to add, "And gain it all back in the next five or ten days!"

But you may be sure of this: When you find the diet which, within the bounds of good health and adequate nutrition, is lower in calories than your energy requirements, you *will* lose weight, steadily, surely, and permanently. No nonsense, no rash promises, no hocus-pocus. Just a consistent weight loss combined with renewed health, an improved appearance, and more vitality.

Easy does it every time. So what's the rush? Let's call it your lifetime eating plan instead of a diet.

Remember that you don't have to settle for a hit-or-miss, up-and-down feast or famine. You can have fool-the-appetite low-calorie feasts that will enable you to get slim— and stay slim.

The 1,400-Calorie Diet
(Basic Menu Outline)

BREAKFAST

Choice of: 1 fruit (high vitamin C fruit such as orange, grapefruit, or strawberries once a day)

2 eggs, poached, boiled, scrambled, shirred (no butter), or 1 egg and 1 ounce of lean meat, or 2 ounces of lean meat (not fried)

1 thin slice of whole-grain bread or toast (if you *must*)

1 tablespoonful of cottage cheese for spread

Black coffee, tea, or Coffee Slim (made with ½ cup coffee and ½ cup hot skim milk), no sugar

Vitamin-mineral food supplement

LUNCH

4 ounces of meat, poultry, or fish, or 1 cup of cottage cheese or yogurt

2 vegetables from Group 1, or 1 vegetable from Group 2 (listed in Chapter 9)

1 low-calorie green or raw vegetable salad

Fresh fruit, gelatin, or junket dessert (made with skim milk and no sugar)

Vitamin-mineral food supplement

DINNER

1 cup of consommé or bouillon

4 ounces of meat, poultry, or fish

2 vegetables from Group 1, or 1 vegetable from Group 2

Tossed green, raw vegetable, lettuce and tomato, or citrus fruit salad

Fresh fruit or low-calorie dessert (recipes in Chapter 15)

Vitamin-mineral food supplement

Limit your liquid intake with meals to one cup of coffee, tea, or Coffee Slim, and one cup of clear broth. Drink as much water or other nonfattening liquids as you please between meals.

No SALAD DRESSING *except:* one teaspoonful of safflower oil and lemon juice for each salad, or one of the low-calorie, high-protein yogurt dressings. See Chapter 14 for these and other recipes.

BREAD ONLY IF YOU ABSOLUTELY MUST; A MAXIMUM OF TWO SLICES A DAY. One slice of whole-grain bread with cottage cheese spread for breakfast and one other meal, but not all three.

No BUTTER ON YOUR VEGETABLES. The secret flavors of herb-seasoned vegetables are discussed later in this chapter.

TRIM ALL FAT FROM MEATS. Broil or roast meat and poultry. Broil, bake, or poach fish.

Midmorning Energizer. Four ounces of tomato juice, mixed vegetable juice, clam juice, or sauerkraut juice fortified with three teaspoonfuls of Brewer's yeast (for extra protein and important B vitamins). Or a cup of consommé with plain gelatin dissolved in it.

Midafternoon Bracer. Tea, coffee, or Coffee Slim. Sweeten with 1 teaspoonful of honey for quick energy, if you wish. Hot consommé or bouillon, or either one on the rocks with a slice of lemon. Your choice of any of the slimming snacks: crisped, raw vegetables, such as celery, radishes, cabbage, cauliflower, raw turnips, cucumber, or carrot sticks. Or a glass of skim milk or buttermilk.

Lullaby Nightcap. Go to bed with a warm, comfortably filled and relaxed feeling by choosing one of these: hot herb tea with honey and skim milk, a glass of buttermilk, hot or cold skim milk, one-half cup yogurt, or hot or cold Coffee Slim made with your favorite coffee substitute for a sleepytime beverage. The calcium in yogurt, buttermilk, and skim milk aids in relieving jangled nerves and inducing sleep. Hot apple juice with a dusting of cinnamon is delicious. Or hot bouillon or consommé, of course. And do try *hot* tomato juice with a sprinkling of celery salt. Have any of them cold if you like, but a warm drink at bedtime is generally more satisfying and relaxing.

If you think that this resembles the Take-Your-Choice Diet, you're quite right. And if you want to take it from here and plan your own menus within this basic outline, I'll consider it a fine idea. Meal planning should be flexible, within calorie limits.

Sample Menus
(Approximately 1,400 calories a day)

BREAKFAST FOR THE WEEK

Begin your day with fresh fruit. An orange, half a grapefruit, or strawberries in season will supply beneficial amounts of vitamin C. Use the basic breakfast menu outline, but vary the eggs and meat to suit your taste. If you like, substitute a bowl of cereal occasionally (not too often, though!) for eggs or meat. *Use only the whole-grain type of cereal found in health food stores—whole wheat, millet, rye, rice, barley, buckwheat, oats, or soy.*

Whole grains of wheat are delicious, soaked overnight and cooked lightly the next morning. Serve topped with a drizzle of honey. You may add one-half cup of skim milk.

Remember, just one slice of whole-grain toast with a tablespoonful of cottage cheese for a spread.

Black coffee, black tea, or Coffee Slim, with no sugar, for breakfast. Also, if desired, for lunch, dinner, and between-meal snacks.

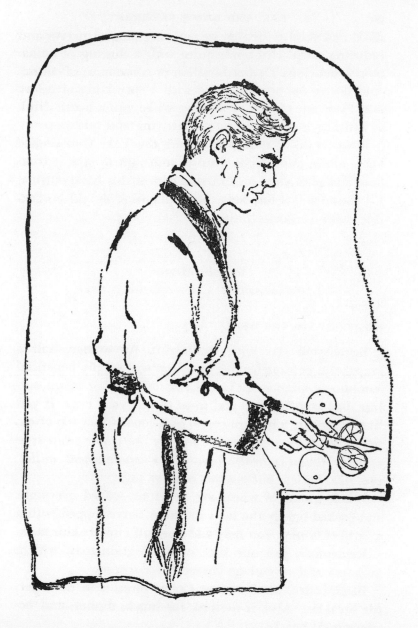

And, for additional nutritional protection, be sure you include a complete vitamin-mineral food supplement.

First Day

LUNCH

Shrimp salad
(½ cup cooked shrimp, ½ cup diced celery, ½ cup diced cucumber. Mix with yogurt Thousand Island dressing and serve on lettuce or other crisp green.)
2 rye or protein wafers, or 1 slice whole-grain bread
1 small slice melon or fresh fruit

DINNER

4 ounces broiled liver
6 stalks asparagus
½ cup cauliflower
Mixed green salad
3 fresh (or unsweetened, canned) apricots

Second Day

LUNCH

1 4-ounce cube steak (simmered in fat-free bouillon)
½ cup broccoli
2 slices tomato on lettuce
½ cup fruit gelatin

DINNER

4 ounces pot roast
½ cup steamed cabbage
Raw vegetable salad
1 slice fresh pineapple with lime

Third Day

LUNCH

4 ounces liverwurst, or broiled liver

Shredded cabbage, carrot, and green pepper salad

2 rye or protein wafers

½ cup junket made with skim milk

DINNER

1 cup consommé

4 ounces broiled hamburger

½ cup stewed tomatoes and celery

½ cup Brussels sprouts

1 fresh fruit cup

Fourth Day

LUNCH

No-Bread Sandwich

(2 ounces cold meat between 2 thin slices of Swiss or Provolone cheese)

1 sliced cucumber on lettuce

1 cup watermelon balls or fresh fruit

DINNER

4 ounces broiled chicken livers

½ cup broiled mushrooms

½ cup broccoli

Mixed green salad

½ cup stewed rhubarb (1 teaspoon honey to sweeten)

Fifth Day

LUNCH

Tuna or salmon salad

(½ cup tuna or salmon—drain off the oil or use dietetic brand—mixed with ½ cup diced celery and ½ cup diced cucumber. Garnish with radish roses and serve on lettuce or other crisp greens. Top with yogurt Thousand Island dressing.)

1 medium apple

DINNER

4 ounces poached, baked, or broiled fish, or crabmeat omelet (2-egg omelet filled with ¼ cup flaked crabmeat)

½ cup winter squash

½ cup spinach or mustard greens

Raw vegetable salad

2 fresh plums

Sixth Day

LUNCH

4 ounces all-beef frankfurter

½ cup sauerkraut

½ cup steamed onions

1 orange or other fresh fruit

DINNER

4 ounces broiled steak

½ cup mushrooms

½ cup green beans

6 celery, carrot, and green pepper sticks

Fruit compote

Seventh Day

LUNCH

Fruit salad
(*Suggestion:* ½ peach, ½ pear, ½ banana, 2 apricots,
and ½ cup grapes. Top with ¼ cup yogurt or with
creamy yogurt dressing.)
2 rye or protein wafers

DINNER

½ chicken, brushed with lemon juice and broiled with
strips of celery over it (no butter)
6 stalks asparagus
½ cup carrots
Shredded cabbage and pineapple salad
½ cup red raspberries or strawberries (a drizzle of honey
to sweeten, if desired)

Your first reaction to this menu pattern may be, "Why,
that's more than I ever eat! How can I lose weight on three
square meals a day?"

It's the only approved, successful way to lose weight, look
better, and live longer. Without a doubt, it's the only
foolproof way to reduce—and *stay* reduced.

Stop and look at the quality of the food instead of the
quantity. Fat-fighting protein and low, low fats, except for
the salad dressing of safflower oil which contains valuable,
fat-emulsifying lecithin, important linoleic acid, and age-
defying vitamin E. It also balances out the *hidden* fats
contained in meat and other food, and works to prevent
cholesterol deposits in the arteries.

The carbohydrate intake consists only of the natural
sugar and starch in vegetables and fruits—unless you insist

on eating the one or two slices of bread a day, and an occasional bowl of whole-grain cereal.

Brewer's yeast, dissolved in juice or skim milk for an energizer or bracer, is loaded with extra B vitamins, including two more fat-dissolving agents, choline and inositol. For added food value, Brewer's yeast may be added to soups, hamburger, or meat leaf.

Still a skeptic? All right, then. Drop down to 1,200 calories a day. One of the easiest and best ways of doing it is simply to cut 200 calories from your basic meal plan each day. But how? And what?

If you've been eating your absolute maximum of two slices of bread a day, that should be the first to go. And stop those wails of wounded protest! What do you want with all that dry stuff, anyway? At 50 (for the very thin slice) to 75 calories a slice—without any kind of spread—do you think it's worth it?

It's no trick at all to cut 200 calories a day from your diet. Deciding what *not* to cut out takes a little figuring. Keep all the protein calories that you can, and eliminate carbohydrates—bread and cereal, even the healthful, whole-grain kind. Look at your fruit and vegetable lists, check the calorie count of each, and substitute low-calorie items for high ones whenever possible. Skip the fruit, gelatin or junket dessert at lunch and save 50 to 75 calories.

I'm in favor of substantial breakfasts when dieting—or at any other time. Maybe you're not. If you're the type who feels pretty noble when you eat breakfast at all, you might save 75 calories by eating one egg instead of two. But, remember, no breakfast-skipping, ever!

To keep from losing weight at the expense of vital tissue, you need protein at each meal, or a total of at least 500 protein calories a day. But on your basic menu you can, with safety, cut your protein for lunch from four to two ounces. You can do it by combining two ounces of shredded meat, poultry, fish, julienne cheese strips, cottage cheese, or yogurt with a big mixed green, combination, or raw vegetable salad. Add a cup of consommé or bouillon, if you wish, and black coffee or tea, and you have a satisfying luncheon of less than 200 calories.

Two eggs, two ounces of hard, *natural* cheese (such as Swiss, Cheddar, or Muenster), ½ cup cottage cheese, or ½ cup yogurt are the equivalent of two ounces of meat and may be substituted for it.

That takes care of the 1,200-calorie diet, easily and safely, too. Just don't cut out *all* the items mentioned. Eliminate two or three things which you will miss the least to total 200 calories, and you have it made.

Sample Menus (900 to 1,000 calories a day)

Don't neglect your energizer of Brewer's yeast and tomato juice (or other low-calorie juice).

Have your protein pickup or nightcap of skim milk, Coffee Slim, buttermilk, or yogurt.

Don't overlook the importance of protecting your body's nutrition at all times—but *especially* while on a reducing program. Include a recommended vitamin-mineral food supplement with each meal.

You *know* the only salad dressings to use—so don't cheat.

Do not snitch a dab of butter, a lump of sugar, or a dash of cream when nobody's looking. The scales are telltales.

BREAKFAST (Basic Plan)

To get the most nutrition in the lowest number of calories, breakfast is standard, or almost. An egg is loaded with protein, vitamins, and minerals. Also that wonder substance, lecithin, abounds in egg yolk—and all for 75 calories. But you have a choice—sort of, anyway.

Choice of: Fresh fruit (or unsweetened, canned, or stewed fruit).

Choice of: 1 egg, poached, shirred, baked, boiled, or scrambled (in a double boiler with skim milk, but no butter). Add 1 tablespoonful cottage cheese, or 1 tablespoonful powdered skim milk, to scrambled egg for additional protein as well as quantity.

Choice of: As a substitute for egg, ¼ cup cottage cheese or ¼ cup yogurt. (Yes, for breakfast—topped with your fresh fruit.)

1 slice whole-grain bread, *if you must,* but no butter.

And, as for all other meals, black coffee, black tea, or Coffee Slim.

First Day

LUNCH

1 cup *hot* tomato juice

Fruit plate

(2 peach halves, 1 cup melon balls, 3 medium apricots. Make substitutions as necessary, depending on availability of fresh fruit. Top with ¼ cup creamy yogurt dressing.)

1 rye or protein wafer

DINNER

4 ounces roast beef

½ cup carrots

½ cup Swiss chard or spinach

Green salad

½ cup applesauce, no sugar

Second Day

LUNCH

2 slices cold roast beef
Cabbage and pineapple salad
¼ cup yogurt dressing

DINNER

1 cup consommé
4 ounces broiled liver
½ cup steamed onions
½ cup green beans
½ grapefruit

Third Day

LUNCH

1 cup sauerkraut juice
1 4-ounce hamburger patty
1 raw tomato
1 slice raw onion

DINNER

4 ounces roast lamb or chicken
2 stalks celery, 2 green pepper rings, and 1 raw carrot
cut in sticks
½ cup broccoli
1 medium pear or apple

Fourth Day

LUNCH

Large green salad
(Combine greens with 2 ounces shredded meat, cheese, or poultry, or two diced hard-cooked eggs—and that's all!)

DINNER

2 medium lamb chops, fat trimmed off
½ cup Brussels sprouts or rutabaga
Raw vegetable salad
½ cup raspberries or blackberries (fresh or frozen)

Fifth Day

LUNCH

1 cup clam broth
½ cup shrimp or crabmeat, or ¼ cup tuna or salmon (with oil drained off) mixed with diced celery and cucumber and marinated with yogurt Thousand Island dressing

DINNER

Broiled or baked halibut or salmon
½ cup cauliflower
½ cup summer squash or ½ small baked potato
Green salad bowl
Small slice honeydew or cantaloupe if in season, otherwise fresh fruit

Sixth Day

LUNCH

½ cup cottage cheese
(mixed with shredded green pepper, raw carrots, and
water cress, topped with 1 tablespoon yogurt dressing)

DINNER

1 cup bouillon
4 ounces broiled steak
½ cup string beans
½ cup Chinese cabbage
Lettuce and tomato salad
1 fruit compote or 1 small slice watermelon

Seventh Day

LUNCH

Shredded cabbage, raw carrot, pineapple, and green
grape salad, with creamy yogurt dressing
2 slices cold meat

DINNER

1 broiled squab or 4 ounces roast chicken
6 stalks asparagus
Mixed green salad
1 banana baked with ¼ cup cubed orange, drizzled with
honey and topped with 1 teaspoon shredded coconut,
or 1 cup strawberries

You may start any meal that you like with fat-free consommé, bouillon, or clam broth, either hot or jellied. Or
have a raw vegetable compote, crisp, colorful, and low-

caloried. Use a glass or crystal dessert dish and slice raw
cauliflower, carrots, tomato, green pepper, celery, cabbage,
or tender, young Brussels sprouts in color-contrasting
layers.

Have celery stuffed with cottage cheese and surrounded
by radish roses for an appetizer any time you like, or serve
your salad first.

You've heard of what happens to the best-laid plans of
mice and men, haven't you? Well, sometimes it happens
to the best-planned diet, too. You lose weight steadily for
a few weeks, and the bathroom scales are your friend:
co-operative, benevolent, kind.

Then—wham!—something goes wrong. The scales go
off their rocker—if they have a rocker. And you almost
go off yours.

You can't seem to lose a pound. Not even an ounce in
a week.

You haven't *looked* at a gooey dessert, or even drooled
over one. What's wrong? You decide that the scales must
be broken. Stuck in that one infernal spot and unable to
budge.

It isn't the scales. It's you. Unfair and unethical as it
seems, it's your bulge that refused to budge.

It isn't according to the rules of the game, I know. It's
a conspiracy, a plot, and it shouldn't happen to anyone.
But sometimes it does happen, so let's face up to it.

You've reached a certain weight plateau. Unreasonably,
unaccountably, in spite of staying on your diet, your lovely
weight loss has leveled off.

What can you do to break the pound barrier?

You can drop down to 750 to 800 calories a day—for four
or five days *only*.

Or you can go on a liquid diet of vitamin-and-mineral-
packed fruit and vegetable juices, plus skim milk protein

pickups, *for one day*. (Two days of liquids are all right if you don't work on those days.)

Another alternative is to eat two regular meals a day (the combined total of *both* meals not to exceed 600 calories) and one meal of the above liquids. (Recipes for liquid meals are given in the next chapter.)

Sample Menus (750 to 800 calories a day)

Absolutely no bread on this diet.

Don't neglect your tomato juice, clam juice, or sauerkraut juice fortified with three teaspoonfuls of Brewer's yeast. Have it either for a midmorning energizer or to start a meal, if you like.

Take your vitamin-mineral food supplements without fail. Care must be taken to obtain all the nutrition possible on any diet, but it's especially important in the lowest caloried meals.

Have your protein pickup or nightcap, as usual, of skim milk, buttermilk, or ¼ cup yogurt. You may have nothing else between meals except slimming snacks of raw vegetables, a cup of consommé or bouillon, or black tea or coffee.

First Day

LUNCH

    1 glass fortified tomato juice, clam juice, or sauerkraut juice (if you didn't have it for your midmorning energizer)

    Large green salad

        (Combine greens with ½ cup diced meat or chicken, and mix with safflower oil and lemon or yogurt dressing.)

DINNER

Broiled liver, average serving
½ cup string beans
Shredded cabbage, carrots, and parsley salad

Second Day

LUNCH

1 medium **tomato,** stuffed with ½ cup cottage cheese,
and garnished with 1 sliced cucumber

DINNER

2 slices pot roast or other lean roast (except pork)
2 oven-browned carrots
2 fresh peach, pear, or apple halves on water cress

Third Day

LUNCH

1 medium hamburger (ground beef patty)
½ cup cauliflower
1 slice raw onion or tomato

DINNER

½ roast or broiled chicken
½ cup spinach or broccoli
1 medium apple or 1 cup strawberries or raspberries

Fourth Day

LUNCH

2 hard-cooked eggs or ½ cup meat, diced, mixed with
tossed salad or lettuce, tomato, celery, shredded carrot, and beets

DINNER

Lean steak, broiled, or cube steak, simmered in bouillon
6 asparagus stalks
½ cup summer squash
3 fresh apricots or 2 plums (fresh or canned)

Fifth (and final) Day

LUNCH

Large green salad mixed with ½ cup dietetic tuna or
salmon or other flaked fish, or ½ cup cottage cheese
with 1 cup fresh berries

DINNER

Any lean fish, broiled, baked, or poached
½ cup mustard greens, spinach, or broccoli
½ cup green beans cooked with mushrooms
Carrot and celery sticks
½ cup rhubarb (sweetened with 1 teaspoon honey) or
½ grapefruit

Have a cup of consommé or bouillon, either hot, jellied,
or on the rocks, to start your meals if you like. The calorie
cost is small for the feeling of satiety given.

You may substitute other fruits and vegetables, with
comparable calorie count, from the groups listed in Chapter 9.

If you prefer to count calories instead of following the
free-wheeling Take-Your-Choice Meals, then do so, by all
means.

But don't ever become a diet bore.

The type who takes along a figurative measuring cup
and calorie chart to consult before each course loses friends

and alienates people. Nobody wants a blow-by-blow account of the bulge in each food binge.

Enjoy your food and let others enjoy theirs.

Count your calories all you like—but not out loud!

Eight Easy Calorie Cuts

1. Always broil, bake, or roast meat and poultry, and broil, bake, or poach fish. For extra flavor with few calories, instead of dotting with butter, baste with tomato juice, bouillon, or a little white wine.

2. If you must eat bread, use a butter substitute of cottage cheese whipped to a creamy spread. Butter has 50 calories per pat, cottage cheese only 15 per tablespoon—and you save at least 35 calories.

3. Budget cuts of meat don't need sauce or gravy to make them appetizing. Try serving them with these low-calorie embellishments: mushrooms (cooked in stock or bouillon, not butter), broiled tomato slices, or strips of braised green pepper and celery with sprinklings of parsley and herbs.

4. Cut your calorie cost in half by getting the habit of substituting skim milk or buttermilk for whole milk. Skim milk, buttermilk, and the ever-handy powdered skim milk contain as much protein and all of the vitamins and minerals (with the exception of vitamin A) that whole milk does, with more than 80 calories saved on each 8-ounce glass.

5. When you fry your breakfast egg it adds up to about 175 calories. Lop off that extra 100 calories by having it poached, boiled, scrambled (in a double boiler with no butter) or baked in a small ramekin or custard cup in 2 tablespoons of skim milk or tomato juice.

6. Pull your figure out of the dumps and boost your energy with another egg idea. Whenever possible, add an extra egg white to your scrambled egg, or combine two or more whites with one whole hard-cooked egg chopped up in a luncheon salad. The white of an egg has only about one-fifth of the calories in a whole egg, but contains more than half of the protein.

7. For the rest of your life skip the sugar-and-starch break of coffee and sweet rolls or doughnuts that most office workers and many housewives have at midmorning or midafternoon, and substitute the healthful, energizing protein pickups, vitamin vitalizers, or slimming snacks.

8. Cut down on meat calories without cutting down on the important protein portions. Simply trim every shred of visible fat from all meat to make sure that it's *really* lean, and see to it that it's cooked *simply* without butter, gravy, or sauce.

How To Season Without Butter

"What about vegetables?" you ask. "They *certainly* have to be seasoned with butter, or they'll taste flat and insipid."

You think so? If you have a taste for the unusual and a flair for the unique, try the following combinations and see how the most pallid, butterless vegetable can become an exotic dish. Remember that all vegetables should be cooked quickly until tender, and not a minute longer.

ASPARAGUS

Cook asparagus whole, or thinly sliced on the diagonal, and season with a bit of salt, freshly ground pepper, snipped chives or chervil, and a few capers. Or if you prefer, try a few drops of lemon juice and a bit of grated cheese. For a dress-up dish, a few almond slivers and a fleck of nutmeg are good.

BEETS

Minced onion and lemon juice zip up the bland flavor of beets. So do caraway seeds, a sprinkle of snipped fresh dill or tarragon, and thyme. Beets can go glamorous with a topping of yogurt, grated orange rind, and allspice.

BROCCOLI

Sautéed minced onion or mushrooms combine well with broccoli, and poppy seeds, curry, tarragon, or marjoram add flavor. If you want to be extra fancy, top with a yogurt-horseradish mixture and shredded raw carrot.

BRUSSELS SPROUTS

Thinly sliced onion, Parmesan cheese, caraway seeds, or sage add flavor. For fanciness combine Brussels sprouts with seedless grapes and a sprinkle of nutmeg.

CABBAGE

Cabbage is good with lemon juice and curry, and better than good with horseradish- or mustard-flavored yogurt, topped with caraway, dill, or celery seed.

CARROTS

Combine carrots with snipped fresh mint, dill, chives, or parsley, or top with a little grated cheese and poppy seeds. Carrots can go slightly exotic with a sprinkle of ginger or nutmeg.

CORN

Cut corn off the cob, add sliced stuffed olives, bits of minced onion, green pepper, or tomato. For corn on the cob, try garlic salt, curry, or brush with chili sauce mixed with celery seed—messy, but good!

GREEN BEANS

Add diced canned water chestnuts, sautéed mushrooms, or scallions to green beans. Flavor with savory, fresh dill, rosemary, or snipped mint. For fun, try a few thin slivers of nuts and a fleck of nutmeg. You might like it!

MUSHROOMS

Fresh or canned, mushrooms are delicious cooked in stock or bouillon with an added dash of sherry. They go well with all other vegetables and add a luxury touch to meat.

ONIONS

Try small whole onions in a sauce of yogurt flavored with soy sauce and caraway seeds. Or slice a large onion and broil with a sprinkle of curry on top.

PEAS

For variety, cook with tiny cocktail onions or diced canned water chestnuts. Curry, savory, or marjoram add flavor, and a few scallions or chives pep them up.

SPINACH AND OTHER GREENS

Zip up greens with safflower oil, lemon juice, and a drop of Worcestershire. Yogurt blended with a dash of horseradish goes well with them. Or moisten with tarragon vinegar to which caraway, poppy, or sesame seeds have been added.

SQUASH, ACORN

Acorn squash is excellent baked with a bit of minced onion and grated cheese. Or for a sweet flavor, bake drizzled with honey and orange juice, with a last-minute dusting of nutmeg.

SQUASH, SUMMER

Soy sauce, a little fresh dill, oregano, or basil will enhance the mild flavor of summer squash. Grated cheese adds a fillip, and so do chopped chives, parsley, and scallions.

TOMATOES

Tomatoes are good broiled with a zippy topping of crumbled Roquefort or blue cheese. For stewed herbed tomatoes, take your choice of fresh dill, basil, sage, marjoram, thyme, or rosemary.

ZUCCHINI

Soy sauce and grated, sharp cheese pep up the bland flavor of zucchini. Basil or marjoram make it flavorful. For a different combination, try zucchini cooked with okra, tomatoes, and minced onion.

There you have them—vegetables seasoned without butter, unique in flavor and low in calories. What's your reason now for not eating to get slim and *stay* slim? You really don't have one left, do you?

Then what are you waiting for? Come on—let's get started!

11

Liquidate That Stubborn Weight

WHAT ABOUT the currently popular commercial food concentrates for liquid diets?

"Nation's Newest Diet Fad Is Just Another Crutch" is the title of a recent article by Dr. Frederick J. Stare, of the Department of Nutrition, Harvard University.

Dr. Stare says that this fad, like the liquid formula diets that were popular a few years ago, simply represents another type of crutch for the overweight to lean on.

When magazine and newspapers published a liquid formula diet featuring dextrose in the not-so-distant past, the results were alarming. Dextrose supplies all over the country were swallowed up almost overnight. One Utah firm which previously sold about sixteen pounds of dextrose every six months began to fill demands for unheard-of amounts up to 1,216 pounds in a single month.

The dextrose rush was on, and Dr. Joseph P. Kessler, Utah's acting State health director, was worried. He sent out a public warning to stay away from trick diets. Fads may come and go, but Dr. Kessler's advice is good at any time.

A day's supply of these new diet concentrates (usually in powder form to be mixed with water) contains 900 calories.

You certainly will lose weight on 900 calories a day, from whatever food source. But how long do you think you would stay on a liquid diet? Long enough for it to do any good, or will it do you harm?

It sounds easy at first, doesn't it? And it is, for a day or two. Maybe even for a week which I doubt. But for a get slim and *stay* slim lifetime eating plan? You know the answer to that. It's a definite, emphatic *no!* The simple fact is, people like to eat, and it's a pleasure which shouldn't be denied weight-watchers or anyone else.

But what would happen if, by some strange and unheard-of quirk, you actually enjoyed drinking your meals instead of eating them? What if you could forget the appetizing flavor and aroma of roast beef, broiled steak or chicken, fresh vegetables and fruits, and be satisfied for weeks with nothing more than three or four glasses of namby-pamby liquid a day? Would that be all right?

Again the answer is an uncompromising *no.*

Even a balanced 900-calorie diet, either liquid or solid, is too low for most adults to stay on for any length of time. And liquid meals, which provide no roughage or bulk to aid elimination, can't be continued indefinitely without causing discomfort or actual harm.

Dr. Stare and I are in complete agreement when he states that, in his opinion, *1,200 to 1,500 calories a day of balanced meals offer the best means of reducing for the typical man or woman.*

"We know of only one way to deal successfully with the problem of overweight," he says. "It is not very complicated or expensive. *Simply eat less, exercise more, and consume a variety of foods to insure good nutrition.*"

"Now, wait a minute," you say. "Weren't you going to

tell me how to liquidate that stubborn weight? And now you're talking against liquid diets. So what *am* I supposed to believe?"

Believe in a variety of foods to insure good nutrition, as Dr. Stare says, and which I have emphatically and consistently advised throughout this book as well as several others.

Believe in substituting plenty of protein and an abundance of vitamin- and mineral-rich fresh fruits, vegetables, and salads for the fattening fifteen.

Believe in the advantages of liquid meals when certain circumstances call for them, which means occasionally but not as a long-term project.

Believe in the safety of dropping down to a liquid meal or two (or for a day or two once in a while) when these conditions make it advisable:

1. To break the pound barrier when you've reached a stubborn weight plateau and it seems as though you'll never lose another pound. Almost all dieters go through this stage, but it passes and you'll start losing again. Dieting is like an obstacle race, and you can help yourself to hurdle this obstacle by a drop in calories for a few days. Several liquid meals won't hurt you.

2. A day of liquid nourishment will give your stomach a rest and help to shed the extra pounds taken on during the holiday season when meals are traditionally (and unfortunately!) heavy, or after a party when you've eaten and drunk more than you should.

3. After dining out and eating every bite of food that's served rather than offend your hostess. Nobody really would have noticed that you didn't (like the Jack Sprats —only there were *two* of them) lick your platter clean of both fat and lean. And you dived right into dessert instead of stalling until it was taken away and contenting

yourself with black coffee. As a result of all this your scales register an honest and unflattering figure.

Instead of rushing out and spending money for prepared commercial products, whip up your own with nonfat milk, fresh fruits and vegetables, and wholesome, unsweetened juices to suit your individual taste and need.

Here are some recipes to get you started. Choose the combinations that appeal to you, or substitute similar mixtures sparked with your own imagination and ingenuity. Powdered skim milk is excellent for protein drinks, and should be on every well-stocked low-calorie shelf.

Vitamin Vitalizers
(These are quick mixes. Simply shake, stir, or whip.)

	APPROXIMATE CALORIES
Grapefruit juice and avocado	95–125

1 cup unsweetened grapefruit juice, ⅛ ripe avocado, mashed.

Pineapple lemonade	100

½ cup pineapple juice, ½ cup lemonade. No sugar. If sweetening is desired use a bit of honey.

Avocado and consommé	95–125

1 cup consommé, ⅛ mashed avocado, chopped chives and pepper.

Tomato juice and sauerkraut juice	45

½ cup each.

Tomato juice and raw onion	50

1 cup tomato juice, 1 teaspoon raw grated onion.

Tomato juice and celery juice   40
½ cup each.

Tomato juice and carrot juice   50
½ cup each.

Orange juice, carbonated water, and fresh mint   50
½ cup orange juice, ½ cup carbonated
water, 2 leaves finely chopped fresh mint.

Papaya juice and pineapple juice   100
Scant ½ cup each.

Tangerine tea   35
1 cup tea, juice of ½ tangerine, 1 teaspoon
honey. Serve hot or iced.

Minted herb tea   40
Choice of herb tea, 1 cup, juice of ½ small
orange, 1 teaspoon lemon juice, 1 teaspoon
honey, sprinkle of powdered ginger. Serve
hot or iced.

Mulled apple juice   85
1 cup hot apple juice, 1 teaspoon lemon juice,
1 clove, light sprinkle of cinnamon.

Red currant and papaya juice   48
¼ cup each. Add 1 tablespoon lemon juice
and fill glass with carbonated water and
crushed ice.

Protein Pickups

(Whatever you do, don't fail to include some of the all-important protein drinks in your liquid diet. Make them of buttermilk, skim milk, powdered skim milk, or yogurt. Include a beaten egg occasionally.)

APPROXIMATE
CALORIES

Tomato buttermilk   60
½ cup buttermilk, ½ cup tomato juice, pinch sea salt, 1 drop Worcestershire sauce.

Buttermilk frosty   90
Freeze ½ cup orange juice to a mushy consistency and mix with ½ cup buttermilk. Vary with ½ cup crushed and semifrozen strawberries for a calorie count of about 65. (Red cherry, apricot, pineapple, peach, and grape juice all combine well with buttermilk, either semifrozen for a frosty drink or mixed in a glass or jar.)

Buttermilk and applesauce   109
½ cup each.

Vegetable buttermilk cocktail   90
1 cup buttermilk mixed with 1 tablespoon shredded cucumber, ¼ teaspoon finely grated onion, 2 teaspoons finely grated celery, 1 tablespoon shredded carrot, ½ teaspoon lemon juice.

Oriental tang   95
½ cup tangerine juice, ½ cup papaya juice mixed with 2 tablespoons of powdered skim milk. Shake until frothy and top with 1 tablespoon finely shredded fresh or water-pack pineapple or a few coconut shreds.

Yogurt red velvet   75
¼ cup yogurt, ¾ cup tomato juice, dash celery salt.

Beet juice and yogurt   95

⅔ cup beet juice, ⅓ cup yogurt, fresh dill.

Yogurt-orange shake   110

¼ cup yogurt, ¾ cup orange juice, dusting
of nutmeg.

Grape milk shake   80

¾ cup skim milk, 1 stiffly beaten egg white,
2 tablespoons grape juice, vanilla or cinnamon to taste.

Coffee milk shake   88

1 cup skim milk, 1 teaspoon instant coffee,
¼ cup carbonated water, ¼ teaspoon vanilla or almond extract. Pour mixture from
one glass to another until it foams, then serve
at once.

Orange milk shake   100

½ cup skim milk, ½ cup orange juice, 1
stiffly beaten egg white, 1 teaspoon grated
orange peel.

Orange-egg cocktail   90

½ cup orange juice, ½ cup carbonated
water, 1 well-beaten egg yolk, dash sea salt,
nutmeg to taste. Other juices, such as pineapple, apricot, blackberry, currant, raspberry, or strawberry, may be substituted for
the above. Make your own combinations to
suit your taste.

If you have an electric blender or juice extractor, your
choice of vitamin vitalizers is practically unlimited. Take
your choice of raw vegetable or fresh fruit combinations
—carrots, tomatoes, celery, green pepper, water cress,

parsley, lettuce, kale, escarole, spinach, mustard, turnip, and dandelion greens—and change thcm almost magically into liquid salads.

The Duchess of Windsor is fond of fresh pineapple blended with water cress. Mitzi Gaynor keeps her figure trim and her energy high with protein pickups of various fresh fruits whipped with cottage cheese to a consistency of malted milk.

Manya Kahn, head of a New York salon which has been dedicated to health and beauty for twenty-five years, is in favor of the easy-does-it diet plan of *no more than one liquid meal a day*. She also advises daily exercise, especially while dieting, to prevent loss of muscle tone and flabbiness.

Miss Kahn has five popular, nutritious recipes for liquid meals, to be mixed in a blender and chilled before drinking. All of them contain protein, in the form of skim milk or eggs, and may be classed as protein pickups which are substantial enough for one liquid meal a day.

1. $\frac{1}{2}$ banana, 1 glass skim milk, $\frac{1}{2}$ cup fresh orange juice.
2. $\frac{1}{4}$ ripe cantaloupe, $\frac{1}{2}$ glass skim milk, $\frac{1}{2}$ cup pineapple juice, preferably fresh.
3. 6 fresh apricots, $\frac{1}{2}$ glass skim milk, 1 egg.
4. 3 fresh peachcs, 2 egg yolks, $\frac{1}{2}$ cup fresh orange juice.
5. 1 ripe peeled apple, 1 egg yolk, 1 glass skim milk.

If you're a busy person (and who isn't?) a liquid meal is a time-saver as well as a calorie-saver. It may be just the time you need to become your own shapemaker.

12

Be Your Own Shapemaker

YOU'VE LOST WEIGHT, you look well, feel wonderful, and have your appetite under control. Still you don't quite stack up to your own satisfaction. What's wrong?

Maybe you haven't lost in the preferred places. You still may have a few undesirable bumps and bulges, or your skin is flabby and lacks tone.

If you kept your diet high in protein, it has aided in better weight distribution and helped to prevent loss of muscle tone and excessive flabbiness.

But if you're one of the many who find it almost impossible to lose weight proportionately, then some form of exercise and spot reducing for the problem areas may be the answer.

Before you shudder at the thought and sink back into the comfort of an overstuffed chair, listen to Terry Hunt, the famous shapemaker of Hollywood stars. "Your weight can be ideal," he says, "but that alone doesn't make the perfect figure. Your tape measure will reveal what's wrong with your shape with far more accuracy than your bathroom scales."

I said earlier that exercise alone won't reduce your weight to any great extent. It won't. Neither will massage. It is estimated that it would take about four hours of strenuous massage—if you could last that long—to get rid of eight ounces. At that, your masseur would lose more weight than you would.

Here's what exercise *will* do. It will firm you up, tone your muscles, redistribute your weight, and shape you to desirable proportions. It will help you to lose in inches, if not in pounds. It will fill in hollows left in your neck, shoulders, and chest, and it will pare down stubborn bulges that dieting alone may fail to budge.

If you're the type who says, "I don't want to lose any more weight in my face, neck, or bust, but I still need to take a few inches off my hips and waist," then exercise is for you.

Moderate exercise is good for almost everybody.

Do you want to be able to wear a bathing suit and be a reasonable facsimile of Esther Williams or Jack La Lanne?

Take a good look at the boys and girls on the beach. Not the lazy sun-bathers on the sand, but the ones who really swim. You won't see any flat chests, thick waists, bulging midriffs, or flabby arms and legs among the swimmers.

Swimming is one of the finest ways to build up or whittle down various parts of the body. The crawl stroke trims the waist and hips, and the backstroke firms flabby arms and muscles. The breast stroke is aptly named. It can reduce or develop (as needed) your chest, shoulders, neck, and rib cage. Swimming uses all of the body muscles and conditions and relaxes you at the same time.

If you can't or won't swim, try dancing, tennis, or bowling, or even a brisk daily walk. Find something that's fun to do, and you'll be more consistent about doing it.

"I never went in for sports," you say, "and I certainly don't have time for them now."

All right. Do you have twenty minutes a day to spend on yourself? Or fifteen? Even ten?

Then take the advice of a man who is an authority on body conditioning. John Dziegiel, athletic trainer at Fordham University and for the New York Giants professional football team, says that there is no reason why any man or woman can't do *some* beneficial exercises.

"The main thing is consistency," he says. "It's not how much you do, but how regularly you do it. *I'd say that if a person did just five sit-ups and five honest, deep-knee bends each and every day, he'd be doing himself a lot of good.*"

He also recommends the old-fashioned bicycle riding exercise.

You might start your day by waking up with the Kitten Stretch.

Of course, if you're a man, you may not like this idea. You'll probably say, "Who does this guy, Kordel, think he is? Does *he* do the Kitten Stretch? It's all right for the girls, but you won't catch *me* doing any such sissy-sounding exercise!"

You don't have to. For the sake of your virility we'll call it something else. It's now the Tiger Stretch, if you choose.

The Take-Your-Choice Stretch—Kitten or Tiger

Upon awakening, rotate your head from side to side, arch your back, and stretch your legs until you feel the pull in the back of your knees. Get up slowly, still stretching arms, legs, and torso, and stand with feet apart.

Raise your arms and stretch them high above your head. Reach higher and higher toward the ceiling until you almost lose your balance. Then lower arms, bend from the waist, keep your knees straight, and touch your fingers to the floor, first in front of you, then on each side, as far back as you can go by twisting at the waist. Repeat the stretching, reaching, bending, and twisting ten times. This is good for circulation, grace, and general limbering up.

Now, while you're as relaxed and comfortable as a kitten or tiger, you might do three minutes of the bicycle exercise, working up to five minutes after a week.

"All this before breakfast?" you ask.

Why not? It takes less than ten minutes to start your day feeling lithe, invigorated, and more alive. Isn't it worth it?

A little more time is involved if you need exercises for problem spots, but you can ease into them gradually and do them at your convenience.

Here, also for your convenience, are some timesaving ways to condition while you concentrate and whittle while you work.

If You Sit at a Desk

That occupational hazard, the middle spread, must be coped with and controlled. Your abdominal cavity is entirely sustained by muscles that form a natural girdle through your middle. When the years and lack of exercise weaken these muscles they become as ineffective as an old, limp, two-way stretch. But unlike a worn-out elastic girdle, your muscle girdle can be strengthened.

1. *Sit tall at your desk.* Slumping crowds your vital organs, deprives you of oxygen, causes a hump of fat to col-

lect on the back of your neck, and contributes to a bulky waist and a paunchy abdomen.

2. *Take up those slack folds of flesh and tighten your muscles by a change of posture.* Pull your waist up out of your hips, your ribs out of your waist, and your neck out of your shoulders by stretching up and out. There, now. Doesn't that pull you out of your slump and into neat, taut lines that make you look and feel more slender?

3. *Flatten your abdomen and get rid of flabbiness.* Still sitting tall, pull in your stomach hard and hold it for the count of ten. (Ex-Marines will remember this effective if inelegant command, "Suck in that gut!") Do this ten times three times a day, and in between times whenever you think of it, until your muscles strengthen, your paunch flattens, and holding a trim, flat line becomes habitual. Vic Obek, athletic director at New York University, says that this can help you take an inch off your waist in a week.

4. *Exercise your neck and shoulder muscles.* Turn your head, not your body, to look out the window, at the filing cabinet, at your secretary, or wherever, and give those tense neck and shoulder muscles a workout. Use the time spent talking on the phone to rotate your head backward, forward, and sideways. Do a deep shoulder shrug that hunches your shoulders up to your ears, then relax and slowly lower shoulders.

5. *Slim your ankles, firm your legs, and stimulate circulation.* Underneath your desk, slowly raise one leg and hold it out straight from the knee, arching the instep and rotating the ankle until you feel the muscles pull in the back of the knee and leg. Slowly lower one leg as you raise the other, with the same arching and rotating process. Then raise both legs together, arch and rotate, and lower slowly to the floor.

6. *Develop and strengthen your chest muscles and firm flabby upper arms.* Place both hands beneath your desk, palms up, and lift—lift hard—as though you were trying to lift the desk off the floor. Relax and repeat several times.

If You're a Housewife

Do the same routines, but in Exercises 5 and 6, instead of a desk, use the kitchen table as you're having your lunch or midday energizer.

"Just when do you think that a housewife gets a chance to sit down to practice the first three?" you ask.

You don't have to sit down to do them. You can do them standing up, as you wash the dishes or iron.

I know one ex-ballet dancer, now a housewife, who has turned her kitchen counter into an exercise bar. She just throws one leg up over the counter (alternating legs) and balances on the other as she washes the dishes.

But if you try it, lose your balance, and break the dishes, don't blame me!

For a foot, ankle, and leg exerciser and a muscle co-ordinator, this same girl stands on tiptoe as she makes the beds, brushes her teeth, combs her hair, and puts on makeup. I'd advise you not to try it while applying mascara.

Now, don't try to tell me that housewives haven't time to do Exercise 4. I *know* that they talk on the telephone.

Have you finished your phone conversations for the day? Then how about getting to work on those overpadded spots?

Hip Tips

1. *The Fanny Walk.* This is one of the best-known and most effective hip reducers. You'll be more comfortable if you wear slacks for this one, for obvious reasons.

Sit flat on the floor, legs stretched in front of you and arms folded across your chest as in "Look, Ma, no hands!" Then wriggle across the carpet on your derrière, shifting from side to side. Five times daily across the room will show an improvement in a month.

2. *The Hip Spanker.* Lie on back, arms out straight from shoulders, knees bent, and feet raised slightly off the floor. Keep arms and shoulders flat on the floor, and with feet still suspended in the air, swing knees from left to right, rolling over fast from one side to the other until your thighs spank the floor hard on each side as you roll. Start with eight hip-spanks and work up to sixteen.

3. *The Hip Nipper.* Kneel on floor with arms reaching toward the ceiling, back straight, and hips tucked in. Slowly lower body and arms until almost—but not quite— sitting on your heels. Hold for ten counts, then slowly raise body to original upright position on knees, with arms reaching again for the ceiling. Repeat ten times.

Middle-Whittlers

These exercises work together to slim your waist and firm and flatten your abdomen.

1. *The Bicycle Movement.* If you've ever exercised at all, you know how to do it. Just lie on your back, put your hands under your hips, lift your legs high, and pedal through the air as though you were riding a bicycle.

"About five minutes a day act as a wonderful conditioner," says John Dziegel.

2. *The Hollywood Fling.* Jim Davies, exercise coach of famous Hollywood stars, gets results with this one.

Stand erect with legs far apart and toes pointing outward, arms stretched out from shoulders in T formation.

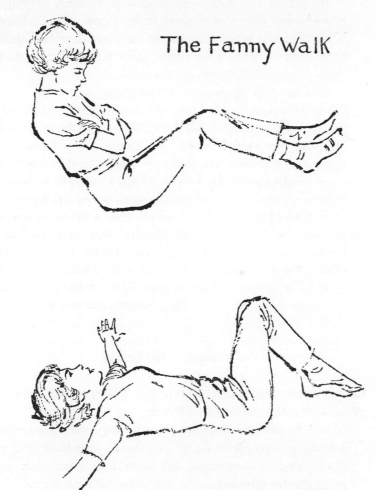

The Fanny Walk

The Hip Spanker

Swing body forward and down, twisting it sideways to bring the right hand across and down to touch left foot. Return to original position. Swing body forward again and twist to opposite side, touching left hand to right foot. Repeat six times.

3. *The Torso Trimmer*. This is hard, but it's a four-way stretch, which slims your waist and hips, firms and flattens your abdomen, strengthens your back, and tones and firms your thighs and legs.

Lie flat on back. Keeping your hips on the floor, slowly raise your upper body and legs simultaneously in the air. Balancing only on your derrière, work to get both head and feet as nearly parallel to each other as possible until your body forms a V shape. Repeat three times, gradually working up to ten.

4. *The Tummy Smasher*. Lie flat on back and pull both knees up to chest. Clasp hands around knees and roll forward to a sitting position, holding back and shoulders straight and head high. Slump and roll back again. Repeat five to ten times.

Bust Beautifiers

1. *Dry Swimming*. The rhythmic action of swimming develops the pectoral muscles that hold up the breasts and make them firm and shapely. If you never go near the water, try swimming, anyway—on dry land.

First, the swimmer's breast stroke, mentioned before.

Sit flat on floor, legs straight in front of you, back straight, chest high, and palms together in front of chest. Shoot arms forward as far as possible in front of you, palms still together. Turn palms out and thrust arms in an arc behind you as far as possible. Then bend elbows and bring arms forward to starting position in front of chest again. This should be done vigorously, so you can feel the pull in chest, arms, shoulders, and back.

Now, the dry land crawl, recommended by Anita Colby.

Lie across the bed, face down, with arms and shoulders suspended free over the edge, arms stretched in front of you. Pull one elbow up out of the "water," slowly reach forward, fingers together, and pull back hard. Roll, and begin the other arm's stroke. Keep one arm following the other in a flow of rolling rhythm. Breathe in deeply on every two strokes, exhaling on next two.

2. *The Push-Pull.* Clasp hands in front of chest, fingers locked together securely. Push palms hard against each other until you feel the pull on underarms and pectoral muscles. Repeat six times and work up to twenty times, after the first few days.

You don't need expensive vibrating tables or belts, massagers, and other gadgets. You can be your own successful shapemaker, and remold your body into lean, lithe lines by your own determination and efforts. Try it and see.

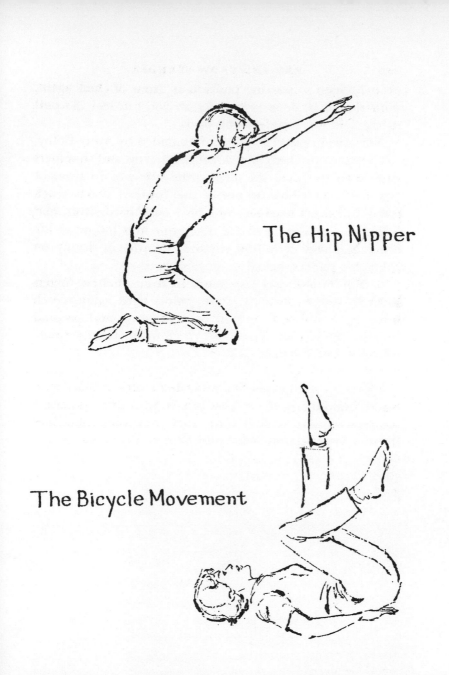

The Hip Nipper

The Bicycle Movement

———————◆———————

13

No Sags, No Bags, No Sad Sacks

BY THIS TIME you should be in fine shape. Middle whittled down and flexible, torso trimmed and firmed, and bulges swapped for lean, neat lines. You can be justly proud of your body.

What about your face? Your chin, throat line, and facial contour? Have you neglected them during your slimming down process and general physical rejuvenation?

Have you kept a young profile?

Are your face and throat line firm and youthful, or do they sag, bag, and otherwise resemble a creased, crumpled, forlorn sad sack? Does your mouth droop at the corners and your chin (I hope it's only *one* by now!) fold into accordion pleats?

What does it profit a person to lose weight and gain sags, bags, and a haggard, lined face and throat?

Let's have none of this unnecessary nonsense! Let's get busy and do something about it.

It would have been better if you had chosen a series of body and facial exercises to fit your needs as you began your reducing program, and proceeded to keep them up for the rest of your youthful-looking life. But you might not have listened to me then. You were intent on reducing, and perhaps exercise didn't occur to you. Like countless others—including myself—you may have to learn the hard way, and repair the damage after it's done, instead of preventing it.

If you *had* been the look-before-you-leap type, you might have listened to this advice. If you combine facial and throat exercises *with your dieting* you won't need to rush into a later program of contour rehabilitation.

No matter what type you are, regardless of age or sex, it's never too late to benefit by following these next suggestions.

1. *Watch your posture and the way you hold your head.* Never, never form the habit of holding your head down with your chin tucked in toward your chest. Even a young, slender person will develop a double chin and a creased jaw line if this way of holding the head isn't corrected.

2. *Hold your head proudly.* Keep your chin up and your eyes high, looking at the stars instead of the gutter.

3. *Remember that your skin needs to be oiled and lubricated while losing weight and afterward.* This is particularly important during sessions of exercise and facial massage. Sesame seed oil, obtainable in health food stores, is an excellent skin softener and sag eraser which is quickly absorbed by the skin. It's easy on the pillowcases and an aid to romance, since husbands—every last man of them!—object to greasy bedtime faces.

If you live alone and are trying to like it, there's no reason why you shouldn't go to bed with night cream on your face and neck if you want to. The experts say that even a dry, thirsty skin will drink in all the oils and moisture possible within twenty minutes, but if you're skeptical (and single) leave it on overnight.

Lubricating creams needn't be expensive. No matter what the advertising claims of high-priced products may be, you can easily mix your own, at a fraction of the cost, which will be just as effective.

Simply take your favorite, inexpensive cleansing cream and mix it half and half with sesame seed oil or pure lanolin. Massage it into your face and throat with light upward and outward strokes, and watch your skin grow smooth and dewy as the oils are absorbed.

Leave it on while you relax in a tub of warm water, and let the heat and moisture speed absorption. Then, speaking for all men, I suggest that you tissue off the excess cream and retire for the night looking rosy, pretty, and lovable.

When morning comes, remember that beauty begins at breakfast. Protein is the master beauty builder and skin firmer, and vitamin B_2 (riboflavin), aided by vitamins A and C, promotes the health of the skin.

Since vitamin C can't be stored by the body, it must be supplied daily. Citrus fruit, as you know, is your best source of vitamin C, and other good sources are strawberries, pineapple, melons, raw fruits, and raw vegetables, especially cabbage and green pepper.

Tomatoes and tomato juice contain some vitamin C, and a considerable amount of vitamin A. Plenty of yellow and leafy green vegetables, liver, and eggs, or capsules of fish liver oil, will insure an adequate vitamin A intake.

If you've been drinking the suggested protein pickups made of powdered skim milk or buttermilk, and the energizers of juice fortified with Brewer's yeast, you've been helping yourself to riboflavin. Many of the foods on your diet menus, including liver, cheese, and broccoli, also supply you with generous amounts of riboflavin, so essential for skin health and beauty.

In his popular column, Dr. William Brady stresses the

importance of riboflavin in maintaining or increasing "the bloom on your cheeks and the sleekness of your skin." He goes on to say that the adult who consumes less than one and one-half pints daily of skim milk, buttermilk, or the equivalent in dry milk powder, is likely to have an unhealthy condition of the skin.

"My skin is healthy enough," you may say. "It should be—I've been following your basic diet plan. There's just too much of it flapping around! I want to know how to take up the slack and lift up the sags."

Let's start with some facial exercises that have been used to firm and tone up the famous faces of many young and not-so-young Hollywood stars.

Face Firmers

1. Jut out your chin as far as you can, raising your lower lip until it covers your upper lip. Tense your muscles, stretch your mouth, and chew hard without touching your teeth together.

2. Same as Exercise 1, except this time press the palms of your hands firmly against your cheeks as you chew hard against the resisting pressure of your hands.

3. Puff out your cheeks, and keep them filled with air as you pat briskly over the laugh lines, out to the ears, and under the chin and jaw line.

4. Stretch your mouth open as wide as you can. Hold your face tense and slowly narrow your mouth into a small O. Then stick your tongue out, as you used to make a face when you were a child. It was naughty then, and it still isn't pretty, but it exercises almost every muscle in your face.

5. Tense your jaw and chin muscles and twist your

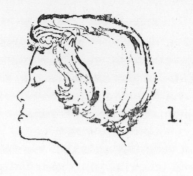

1.

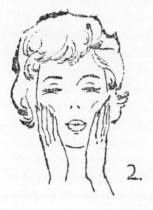

2.

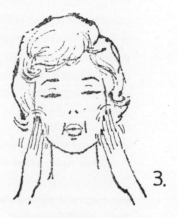

3.

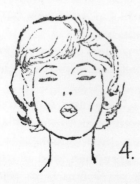

4.

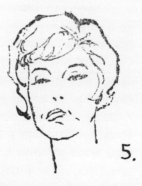

5.

The Face Firmers

mouth far to the right, and then to the left, as though you were talking out of the corner of your mouth.

The muscles in a man's face are not as likely to grow slack and flaccid as those of a woman's. Watch your husband (or father or brother) twist his mouth and chin from side to side as he's shaving, and you'll see the reason for it—and perhaps work out a new routine of facial exercises for yourself.

Lubricate your face and throat with sesame seed oil or your oil and cream mixture, and do these exercises for two or three minutes—later working up to five minutes—every night and morning.

Don't lug around an old neck on your slim, young-looking body. The face firmers are chin and neck firmers, too, but the skin of the neck is thin and needs special attention.

Use your sesame seed oil to smooth away lines and massage a crepey, slack neck into firmness. Rotate your fingers vigorously over the back of the neck where tension gathers, and squeeze and knead the muscles across the top of your shoulders.

A gentle touch is needed for the delicate muscles at the sides of your neck and for your throat. Stroke upward in light, rotary movements from chest to chin, from shoulders to ears, and sideways from chin to ears.

If you have a slant board, or an old ironing board which can be propped up against something to support your weight, ten minutes a day in an upside-down position discourages down-drooping lines. This position improves the circulation of blood to your face, neck, and scalp, and helps maintain contour.

But if you don't have a slant board and your ironing board is built into the wall, then you're just the person for whom I've been saving this extra-special stimulator, exerciser, and contour lift.

The Upside-down Face, Chin, and Neck Lift

Lie flat on your back across the side of your bed, with your head and neck hanging down over the edge. Hang down lower, lower—until the weight of your head pulls the kinks out of your neck muscles. Let your head hang down for a full minute, until you feel the flow of circulation in your face. Then very, very slowly, shoulders still flat on the bed, raise your head and neck straight up to a "sitting" position and rotate from side to side. Hold neck and head erect for a count of ten, then slowly lower them down over the edge of the bed again. You can feel the tremendous muscle pull as you do these neck and chin sit-ups.

Two or three times a day are enough for this one until your neck muscles strengthen, which should be in a week or so. It's a firm, attractive neck that you want—not a stiff one—so use discretion.

You *can* undouble your chin, firm a sagging contour, and keep a young profile. You can do it yourself, without expensive emollients, salon treatments, masseurs, or other outside help. All it takes is a good lubricating oil, a little bit of time, a moderate amount of know-how, and a lot of determined, persistent effort. (Remember sesame oil.)

It's *your* face and neck, the only ones you'll ever have. Your own efforts may determine whether you'll be a vision, or a sight—whether you'll keep a young profile, or let the sags and bags defeat you.

What are you going to do about it?

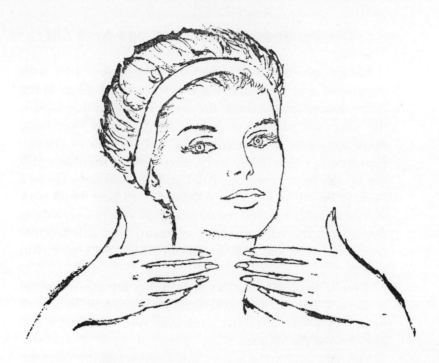

14

Your Eat-for-a-Treat Bonus

IT'S A BAD DAY at Dietsville.

One of those days that can happen to anyone. Your morale is low, and you have an almost uncontrollable desire to go on a reckless food binge.

What can you do? You've been eating to beat the pounds and you've won—temporarily. But you know only too well that you can quickly eat them right back on again.

Once more you have a choice. And there's a bulge in that binge unless you choose wisely. You can do one of several things.

You can give yourself one day—*just once in a while*—to eat the forbidden food that you think you're craving. The chances are that when you try it you'll find out for yourself that none of the fattening fifteen tastes as good as it used to.

Since cutting down on fats, sugar, and starches, your taste buds have become more sensitive and your appetite has been re-educated.

You've become a gourmet instead of a gourmand.

But if you have to prove it to yourself, go ahead and give yourself a day to eat as you please.

Is it rich, goopy desserts that you've missed? Have anything you want—again I say, *for one day*—then go back to your basic diet plan. See how much better you feel, and how good, by comparison, the natural, wholesome flavor of fresh fruit, cheese, melon, berries, or fruit compote tastes.

After your binge, look closely and you can see how even one day of high-carbohydrate food can dull your eyes and dim the radiance of your skin.

Maybe it's an Italian dinner that you crave—a heaping plate of spaghetti with meat sauce and thick slabs of crusty bread slathered with garlic butter. Then have spaghetti. But make it at home. There are several companies that manufacture high-protein spaghetti and macaroni which have a fairly low starch content and a protein content of 20 to 35 per cent. One of these companies has factories in New York, Jersey City, France, and Italy. Their products are usually obtainable in health food stores, or your favorite market can get them for you.

Or instead of spaghetti, wouldn't you like to try some typical Italian meals which Americans never think of as being Italian—high-protein, low-calorie, eat-for-a-treat dishes straight from famous restaurants in Florence and Milan? Then walk with me in Florence, Italy, down a narrow street parallel to the Arno River, on past Ponte Vecchio, until we come to a small, unpretentious restaurant called Camillo's.

Bruno Maisero, the manager of Camillo's, describes his favorite customer as a person with an inner disposition for food *who is perishing for some one special dish.*

That's you, isn't it?

So come and share with me an eat-for-a-treat Italian chicken dinner which is well within your calorie limits. Signor Maisero suggests a white Chianti, Arbia, to go with it. "Arbia has the character to stand up to this dish," he says.

If you can't join me at Camillo's (I wish you *could*), it's a gourmet meal that's easily made at home.

Remove all bones except one from chicken breasts (two breasts for each serving). "Leave one bone so anyone can see it's chicken," says Bruno Maisero. Pound the chicken flat and brown in a small amount of safflower oil, then place in a casserole, garnish with wafer-thin truffles, and sprinkle with Parmesan cheese. Add a few tablespoonfuls of chicken broth, cover the casserole, and finish cooking in the oven.

You don't have to grow your own truffles in your back yard. Get them already grown and in cans at the better food shops.

But if we *should* happen to be in Italy at the same time, let's go on to Milan. Dine with me at Savini's, one of Milan's most elegant restaurants, not far from the famous opera house, La Scala.

And, please, *don't* order spaghetti!

Let the director of Savini's, Angelo Pozzi, suggest the menu. One of my favorite meals at Savini's is simple enough to prepare at home.

First, an antipasto of raw, red mushrooms from Liguria (or your local market), sliced thin and laced with slivers of crisp celery. Sprinkle with Parmesan, or shreds of your favorite cheese, and a bit of lemon juice for dressing. Delicious, and low—*very low*—in calories.

Our main course will be Savini's special fillet of beef, cooked with a sprig of fresh rosemary. A bit of mustard, a tiny dash of cognac, and a drop of Worcestershire sauce may be added to yours just before serving. I prefer mine plain.

For dessert Signor Pozzi suggests fresh red raspberries, if

they're in season, topped with a spoonful of frozen raspberry juice.

No out-of-season foods are served at Savini's. "God made the seasons, and I respect them," Angelo Pozzi says. "Anyway, out-of-season foods are never first-rate."

This is your eat-for-a-treat bonus meal, so if you'd like a glass of wine it's within calorie bounds. Rosé wine from Lake Garda—Chiaretto del Garda—is excellent with a dinner such as ours.

"But I'm like the title of Bob Hope's book," you say. *"I never left home."*

Do you have Chinese, Japanese, or Polynesian restaurants in your home town? Some of the best and most exotic Oriental dishes are fine for reducers and those who want to stay reduced. Their vegetables are lightly and crisply cooked, no fat except a minimum of oil is used in preparing food, and soy sauce is one of their principal seasonings. If there are no such restaurants near you, why not learn the art of cooking delicious, nonfattening Oriental meals yourself?

Let Robert Kawashima tell you how he prepares sukiyaki in his popular Japanese restaurant, Miyako Sukiyaki, in Pasadena, California. "I use the following ingredients to serve four people," he says:

Robert Kawashima's Sukiyaki

1½ pounds top sirloin or rib steak, sliced wafer thin
1 cup celery slices
2 bunches green onions, cut 2 inches long
½ cup sliced fresh mushrooms
½ of a No. 2 can of bamboo shoots, sliced
1 pound fresh bean sprouts
1 cup onions, sliced
1 bunch partially boiled spinach, cut 2 inches long

Preheat an iron pan or 12-inch skillet, coat it with saf-flower oil, and add vegetables, keeping them in separate groups. Add meat and Sukiyaki Cooking Sauce (see recipe below). Turn vegetables and meat over once during cooking. Serve with brown rice, while vegetables are still crisp. Cooking time about 15 minutes.

Sukiyaki Cooking Sauce

2 ounces Japanese wine, sake, if obtainable (if necessary, substitute your favorite cooking wine)

2 teaspoons honey

1 teaspoon monosodium glutamate

½ cup Japanese soy sauce

½ cup consommé or beef stock

Heat all ingredients until thoroughly blended.

The Chinese have a saying that describes a lovely, slender woman. They call her "A woman as lithe and lean as a willow who will sway in the breeze."

It was probably this saying that inspired San Francisco's famous Trader Vic to compile a list of menus for *Harper's Bazaar* called "The Chinese Willow Wand Diet."

The Chinese Willow Wand breakfasts, like my own basic menus, always include fresh fruit rather than fruit juice, and feature an egg, poached, boiled, scrambled (in a double boiler with a bit of parsley), or shirred. The only desserts allowed in the entire ten-day diet are these: sliced orange, small serving lemon sherbet with a squeeze of fresh lemon, two fresh plums, whole stemmed strawberries, melon balls with raspberries, wedge of fresh pineapple, small slice watermelon, ½ cantaloupe, fresh nectarine, fresh raspberries, fresh peach, ½ papaya, fresh pear, ¼ of a 5-inch honeydew melon, and a fruit compote of fresh raspberries, sliced orange, and sliced banana.

No bread is allowed on the diet, except on one solitary breakfast there is a single piece of toast, almost as if it got there by mistake. Another breakfast consists of a hard-cooked egg in $\frac{1}{4}$ cup soy sauce—if you care to try it! Who knows? You might acquire a taste for it.

It's a good diet, with protein and fresh fruit for every meal, although you might get a little tired of Chinese food before the ten days are up.

Except for the use of rice, which is not for the weight-watcher—Oriental cooking is low in calories. (Generally speaking, of course, because there are exceptions!) Their use of fat is confined almost exclusively to a small amount of vegetable oil. Their vegetables are cooked lightly and crisply—never overcooked—and retain a good deal of valu-abel natural vitamin and mineral content.

Below, as an added eat-for-a-treat bonus, are some easily-prepared Oriental recipes which have been adapted for home use from the Chinese Willow Wand Diet. You'll find them to be slenderizing good eating.

Lobster, Chinese Style

2 1-pound lobsters, **split** lengthwise
2 tablespoons soy sauce
1 teaspoon sherry

1 small onion, finely chopped
2 tablespoons water

Steam lobsters over boiling water. When cooked, split lengthwise. Mix together the soy sauce, sherry, onion, and water, and pour it on each $\frac{1}{2}$ lobster. Steam 10 minutes longer. (Serves 4.)

Beef Fugi

1 pound fillet or sirloin
    steak
½ cup mushrooms
2 stalks celery
4 onions
¼ pound Chinese peas
    (snow peas)
½ pound bamboo shoots
12 water chestnuts

Safflower oil
Salt, pepper, and monoso-
    dium glutamate to
    taste
½ cup consommé or chic-
    ken stock
Vegetable thickening or sun-
    flower seed meal
High-protein noodles

Shred meat and vegetables julienne style. Chinese peas
are to be cut in long slivers, pod and all, using sharp knife.
Sauté the beef in safflower oil, then salt and put aside.
Sauté vegetables, add ½ cup consommé or chicken stock
and cover tightly until it boils. Add beef, seasoning, and
thicken with vegetable thickening or sunflower seed meal.
Serve with low-calorie, high-protein noodles, obtainable at
health food or fancy food stores. (Serves 4.)

Broiled Soya Chicken

2 chickens, split in half
2 cups soy sauce
1 teaspoon dry mustard
2 cloves garlic, minced

1 teaspoon powdered
    ginger
½ cup sherry

Marinate chicken in sauce made of ingredients above for
at least ½ hour, turning several times. Then broil, basting
frequently with the sauce. (Serves 4.)

Hamburger, Chinese Style

2 pounds ground round
    steak
20 water chestnuts, finely
    chopped
2 medium-sized onions,
    finely chopped

Salt, pepper, and monoso-
    dium glutamate to
    taste
2 tablespoons oyster or soy
    sauce
4 egg yolks

Mix ground meat with chopped onions, water chestnuts, seasonings, and egg yolks. Shape into patties and broil. (Serves 4.)

Chinese Beef with Peppers

Sauté 1 crushed garlic clove in safflower oil. Remove garlic and add 1 pound lean beef sliced very thin. (Use sirloin, round, chuck, or other lean portions of beef; Chinese cooks vary meat cuts, depending on current prices, availability, individual taste.) Sauté a few minutes. Add 1 cup chopped green pepper, 1 teaspoon powdered ginger, and sauté a minute longer. Add 1 cup hot soup stock, let simmer a few seconds, then add 1 tablespoon soy sauce and thicken with vegetable thickening or sunflower seed meal. (Serves 4 to 6.)

Cabbage, Chinese Style

Sauté 1 cup each shredded cabbage, chopped celery, sliced green pepper, and chopped onion in 1 tablespoon safflower oil, stirring constantly. Add 1 cup chicken broth and steam 2 minutes. Use Chinese cabbage whenever available, it is more delicious. (Serves 4.)

Bean Sprouts with Celery

Sauté 3 stalks chopped celery, 1 small chopped onion, and 6 sliced mushrooms in safflower oil. Add 1 pound bean sprouts, 1 tablespoon each soy sauce and water, salt and monosodium glutamate to taste. Let simmer 5 minutes, stirring frequently. (Serves 4.)

Shrimp Foo Yong

4 eggs	4 tablespoons Chinese peas
4 tablespoons chopped bam-	(snow peas) cut in
boo shoots	long strips
4 tablespoons chopped	½ cup finely chopped
water chestnuts	shrimp
2 cups bean sprouts	Safflower oil

Mix all the chopped vegetables and shrimp and fold in the beaten eggs. Sauté in safflower oil about 5 minutes. (Serves 4—and *no* sauces or gravies, please!)

Would you like to try a variation of a Javanese recipe that won $10,000 in the Henry Kaiser Cook-Out contest? The original recipe is by Bob Gribbroek. I've modified it to lower the calorie cost and to fit your needs. It's now a $9,998 recipe.

Beef Tenderloin, Javanese

Cut 2 pounds beef tenderloin in 1-inch slices across the grain. Marinate the beef in a sauce made of the following for at least one hour:

¼ cup safflower oil	1 cup onion, minced
2 tablespoons honey	2 cloves garlic, minced
2 tablespoons ground coriander	6 Brazil nuts, grated
¼ cup soy sauce	¼ tablespoon dried ground chili peppers
¼ cup lemon juice	

Skewer the beef slices horizontally, with grain facing up. If you have a barbecue, grill over coals 10 minutes on each side. If not, broil 10 minutes on each side. Baste with sauce once on each side during cooking. Serves 4 to 6—with one of the following vegetables:

Savory Sauerkraut

1 apple, cored, peeled, and chopped	1 cup yogurt
1-pound can sauerkraut	½ tablespoon caraway seeds
3 tablespoons tomato sauce	2 tablespoons honey
1 tablespoon onion, chopped	¼ tablespoon salt

Drain excess juice from sauerkraut, place in mixing bowl, and stir in other ingredients, blending well. Put mixture in casserole which has been lightly coated with safflower oil. Bake 20 minutes in moderate oven. (Serves 4 to 6.)

Epicurean Eggplant

1 large eggplant	1 tablespoon onion, finely
1½ teaspoons salt	chopped
¼ teaspoon ground black	½ cup yogurt
pepper	Paprika
	Parsley

Peel eggplant and cut into ½-inch slices and then into cubes. Place in saucepan with ½ inch of boiling water and 1 teaspoon of the salt. Cover and cook 4 to 5 minutes until cubes are tender but still retain their shape. Drain. Add remaining salt, pepper, onion, and yogurt. Heat, but do not boil, until yogurt is hot. Garnish with paprika and parsley. (Serves 4 to 6.)

Everybody knows that salads are chock-full of vitamins and minerals, from the simplest tossed greens to the most spectacular super-concoction. And almost all of them are fine for weight-watchers.

But don't fall into a salad trap. All that glistens isn't a low-calorie green. It may be that those gleaming greens are drenched in French dressing. Or even worse, mayonnaise or Thousand Island dressing.

Suppose that you're having a salad for luncheon. That's all you're going to eat, and you're hungry, so you decide to make it a substantial one. You remember that you need protein at each meal. (I'm proud of you for that, anyway.) But then you go completely overboard.

You eat a small avocado stuffed with shrimp and topped with a mound of mayonnaise. You do it without counting the cost or the calories, and you feel pretty virtuous because you had nothing but a salad and black coffee.

All right. Now, let's go back and figure it up. A small

avocado, 425 calories (honestly!), ten average shrimps, 100 calories, a mound of mayonnaise—say three tablespoons— 300 calories.

Your salad and black coffee add up to an appalling total of 825 calories!

Next time, even on a food binge, stop and take stock just a little. Not enough to take the joy out of it, but to remember and apply the rule of substitution.

Substitute a fresh medium-sized tomato (25 calories) for the avocado and save 400 calories on that alone. Or half a papaya, if you want an unusual delicacy, has a calorie count of 60 to 70, depending on size. It combines well with shrimp, crabmeat, or lobster for a gourmet salad.

By substituting a low-calorie salad dressing you can make your most sensational calorie saving. Regular French dressing, mayonnaise, or Thousand Island dressing average 100 calories a tablespoonful. Here are my recipes, which contain a minimum of 3 calories and a maximum of 14 for each tablespoonful.

French Dressing Substitute
(3 calories per tablespoon)

½ cup tomato juice
¼ cup wine or cider
   vinegar

1 tablespoon onion, finely
   minced
Salt and pepper

Mix all ingredients and shake well. Makes about ¾ cup. Store in refrigerator.

Yogurt Mayonnaise
(11 calories per tablespoon)

1 egg yolk
¾ cup yogurt
½ teaspoon dry mustard
¼ teaspoon salt

Pinch cayenne pepper
Pinch paprika
1 tablespoon wine or cider
   vinegar

Beat egg yolk well and combine with other ingredients until well mixed. Makes about 1 cup. Store in refrigerator.

Yogurt Thousand Island Dressing
(14 calories per tablespoon)

1 cup yogurt mayonnaise
(see recipe above)
1 hard-cooked egg, chopped

1 teaspoon pimiento, chopped
1 teaspoon onion, minced
2 tablespoons chili sauce

Mix all ingredients well and chill before serving. Makes about 1 cup. Store in refrigerator.

Tangy Yogurt Dressing
(10 calories per tablespoon)

1 cup yogurt
¼ teaspoon each of garlic powder, paprika, caraway seeds (whole or crushed)

½ teaspoon parsley, chopped
Salt and pepper to taste

Mix seasonings into yogurt and blend thoroughly. Cover jar tightly and chill 8 hours or more before use. Makes 1 cup.

Creamy Fruit Dressing
(11 calories per tablespoon)

1 cup yogurt
3 tablespoons pineapple or orange juice

1 teaspoon honey
¼ teaspoon cinnamon
⅛ teaspoon mace

Blend together well and keep in refrigerator. Makes 18 tablespoons. Excellent with fruit salads.

Other eat-for-a-treat bonus meals which are low in calories (some are not so low in price, but these are suggestions for your food binge without bulges, not your basic menus) include the following:

	APPROXIMATE CALORIES
Clams Casino (sprinkled with chopped onion, green pepper, and pimiento, broiled. 6 clams.)	75
Deviled crabmeat (mixed with egg yolk, minced onion, green pepper, and Parmesan cheese.)	180
Smoked oysters (5 medium size)	100
Broiled shad roe	170
Broiled soft-shelled crabs	125
Broiled brook trout (with lemon sauce)	100
Broiled lobster	200
Broiled South African lobster tail	120
Broiled sweetbreads	175
Roast pheasant	175
Broiled quail	150

Yes, I know. I warned you, didn't I? You don't make a habit of munching on pheasant, quail, or South African lobster tails. These are for the occasional bonus meal that can be both colorful and low-calorie.

You don't have to make dieting a grim business. I want you to believe that there is a pleasant, satisfying way to reduce and *stay* reduced. You can enjoy gourmet meals and lose weight while you're doing it.

"But it's desserts that are my downfall," you say. "Me and my uncontrollable sweet tooth! What am I going to do about that? You haven't given us any desserts except fruit."

That isn't an oversight. But you always save dessert until last, don't you? At least I hope you do.

In the next chapter you'll find recipes for nonfattening desserts and other suggestions on how to eat and *stay* slim.

15

Delicious Desserts Without Sugar

A FRIEND OF MINE once told me, "One of my great pleasures is taking beautiful women out to dine—in fact, you might call it my hobby. But I feel very bad when I think of some of the charming creatures that I've known and loved, and wined and dined."

"Why? What happened to them?" I asked.

"They ate too much," he said. "They could resist everything—except food. Unlike the true gourmet, they weren't content merely to taste and savor. They ate every bite that was served them. They gobbled and grew fat. And of course their loveliness vanished in a sea of temptation, tallow, and tubbiness."

The mixed metaphor is his, not mine. But he made a good point. If some forbidden delicacy tempts you, taste and savor if you like. *Don't gobble and grow fat.*

"That might work with some people," you say, "but not with me—especially with any kind of sweet. The more candy and cake I eat, the more I crave."

That can easily happen to the person who fails to eat enough protein. And there's a simple explanation for it.

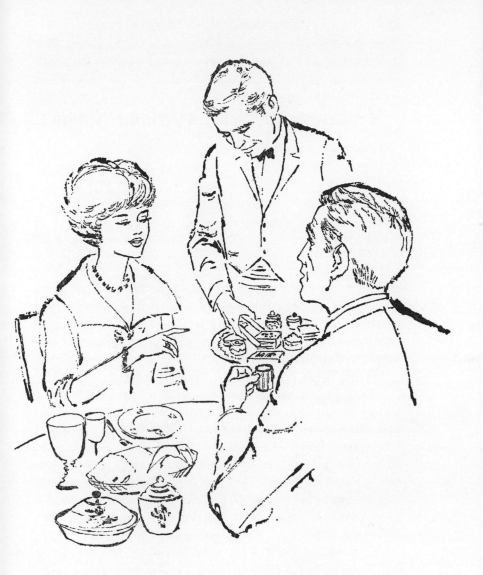

Sugar forces a rapid rise in your blood sugar, which in turn stimulates the secretion of insulin to take care of the sugar. Sugar burns quickly, and after its sudden rise your blood sugar zooms down almost immediately to a new low which causes fatigue and an unsatisfied hunger. Protein foods protect you from this type of craving. Protein three times a day (don't forget a high-protein breakfast) keeps your blood sugar on an even level, neither letting it rise high enough to overstimulate nor sinking low enough to cause a hunger rebound.

I know I promised some desserts, but I *didn't* promise you sugar. Nor did I promise you any concoctions made out of the terrible trio: fats, white flour, and sugar.

And here they are. Desserts without sugar. Sweet-tasting, nonfattening, delicious, and healthful. I hope you like them.

Neapolitan Biscuit Tortoni
(About 55 calories per serving)

3 tablespoons lemon juice
¾ cup cold water
½ cup skim milk powder
3 teaspoons honey
¼ teaspoon vanilla
Dash of almond extract

Pour lemon juice and water in mixing bowl and add skim milk powder. Beat with a rotary beater until stiff. Then add honey, vanilla, and almond extract. Beat again until well blended. Pour into individual cups. Place in refrigerator and freeze as fast as possible, with refrigerator turned to highest point. Serve frozen. (Serves 6.)

Pineapple Yogurt Sherbet
(About 100 calories per serving)

1 cup yogurt
1 tablespoon lemon juice
½ cup pineapple juice
  (unsweetened)
¼ cup crushed fresh or
  frozen pineapple
1 tablespoon honey
2 egg whites

Mix yogurt, lemon juice, pineapple juice, pineapple, and honey thoroughly. Put in freezer tray and freeze until firm. Then take it out, put in a bowl and stir until mixture is smooth and free of lumps. Beat egg whites until stiff and fold them into the smooth, creamy mixture. Return to freezer tray and freeze. (Serves 3.)

Orange Sherbet
(About 82 calories per serving)

1½ teaspoons plain gelatin
¾ cups water
2 tablespoons honey
¼ cup fresh skim milk
1½ cups orange juice

2 tablespoons grated orange rind
1 teaspoon lemon juice
2 egg whites, stiffly beaten
Pinch of salt

Dissolve gelatin in ¼ cup cold water. Bring ½ cup water to boil. Add honey and boil 5 minutes. Add milk and gelatin. Mix well. Remove from heat. Add orange juice, orange rind, lemon juice, salt. Stir well. Pour into freezer tray and set control at level recommended for freezing ice cream. Chill until mixture starts to thicken. Remove to chilled bowl and beat with rotary beater until mushy. Fold in stiffly beaten egg whites. Return to freezer tray and chill until firm. (Serves 6.)

Apricot Sherbet
(About 70 calories per serving)

1½ pounds ripe apricots
1½ pints water
3 tablespoons honey

1 cup fresh skim milk
Juice of 1 lemon
Juice of 1 orange

Wash and pit apricots. Boil water and honey slowly in saucepan for 5 minutes. Press apricots through a sieve into mixing bowl. Slowly blend apricot pulp, boiled sweetened water, skim milk, and orange and lemon juice. Press through sieve again. Pour into freezer trays and place in refrigerator. When it begins to freeze around the edges, pour into chilled bowl and beat with rotary beater until smooth. Return to freezer trays until frozen and ready to serve. (Serves 6.)

Low-Calorie Vanilla Ice Cream
(About 80 calories per serving)

2 cups double-strength skim milk (use 1/4 cup skim milk powder to make 1 cup)
3 tablespoons honey

1 1/2 teaspoons vanilla
1 envelope unflavored gelatin
1 tablespoon cold water

Place double-strength skim milk, honey, and vanilla in saucepan. Heat over low flame until just warm, not hot. Remove from heat. Dissolve gelatin in cold water, add to warm milk, stir until well mixed, and pour into freezer tray. Let stand at room temperature for about 10 minutes. Place in freezer unit of refrigerator and turn dial to highest point. Freeze until firm, remove from tray to chilled bowl and beat until smooth. Return to freezer tray and freeze until ready to serve. (Serves 6.)

Low-Calorie Coffee Ice Cream
(About 80 calories per serving)

Same recipe as above, but add 2 tablespoons instant powdered coffee to warm milk mixture. (Serves 6.)

Chocolate Chiffon Dessert
(About 100 calories per serving)

Use carob powder, which looks and tastes like chocolate, when you crave a chocolate dessert. It's low in starch, rich in calcium and natural sugar, and has only 2 per cent fat. (Chocolate has 52 per cent fat.)

1 envelope unflavored
    gelatin
4 tablespoons honey
¼ teaspoon salt
⅓ cup carob powder

3 egg yolks
1½ cups fresh skim milk
1 teaspoon vanilla
3 egg whites

Mix together gelatin, honey, salt, and carob powder in top of double boiler. Beat egg yolks, combine with skim milk, and add to gelatin mixture. Cook over boiling water, stirring constantly until gelatin is thoroughly dissolved, about 5 minutes. Remove from heat. Add vanilla. Chill until it starts to thicken. Beat egg whites until stiff and fold in gelatin mixture. Turn into individual molds and chill until firm. Unmold and serve with Fluffy Mocha Topping, if desired. (Serves 8.)

Fluffy Mocha Topping
(About 23 calories per serving)

¼ cup ice water
¼ cup dry skim milk
¼ teaspoon vanilla

2 teaspoons honey
1 teaspoon instant coffee

Beat together ice water and powdered milk with a rotary beater until mixture is stiff and stands in peaks, which will take about 10 minutes. Then gradually beat in vanilla, honey, and instant coffee. Makes one cup of the topping.

Pineapple Graham Cracker Cake
(About 110 calories per serving)

1 envelope unflavored
    gelatin
1¼ cups canned, crushed
    pineapple (unsweet-
    ened) and juice
3 tablespoons honey
¼ teaspoon salt

3 egg yolks
1 tablespoon lemon juice
3 egg whites
½ cup ice water
½ cup dry skim milk
    powder
6 graham crackers

Mix together gelatin, crushed pineapple and juice, honey, and salt in top of double boiler. Beat egg yolks lightly. Add to gelatin mixture and cook over boiling water, stirring constantly, about 8 minutes, until gelatin is dissolved. Remove from heat. Add lemon juice and chill until it begins to thicken. Beat egg whites until stiff and fold in gelatin mixture. Beat skim milk powder and ice water until it stands in peaks, and fold into gelatin mixture. Spoon one fourth of mixture into 9″ x 5″ loaf pan. Top with two graham crackers. Repeat twice to form 3 graham cracker fillings, and top with final layer of the chiffon mixture. Chill until firm. (Serves 8.)

Baked Custard
(About 65 calories per serving)

2 cups fresh skim milk	1 teaspoon vanilla
2 eggs	¼ teaspoon nutmeg or
1 tablespoon honey	cinnamon
¼ teaspoon salt	

Scald milk in top of double boiler over boiling water. Beat eggs until frothy, stir in honey, salt, and vanilla. Add hot milk and mix well. Strain into individual custard cups. Sprinkle with nutmeg or cinnamon. Set the filled cups in pan of hot water with water reaching to approximately ½ inch to top of cups. Bake in slow oven (300 degrees) 1 hour, or until knife inserted in custard comes out clean. Top with low-calorie "whipped cream" made with skim milk powder, if desired. (Serves 5.)

Pumpkin Custard
(About 75 calories per serving)

1½ cups canned pumpkin	½ teaspoon vanilla
1½ cups fresh skim milk	1 teaspoon cinnamon
2 eggs	½ teaspoon ginger
2 tablespoons honey	¼ teaspoon salt

Place the pumpkin in a large mixing bowl. Combine milk, eggs, honey, vanilla, cinnamon, ginger, and salt. Add to pumpkin, blending well. Pour into 6-ounce custard cups and bake in moderate oven (350 degrees) 50 to 60 minutes, or until knife inserted in center of custard comes out clean. (Serves 6.)

Eggnog Chiffon Pudding
(About 90 calories per serving)

1 envelope unflavored
   gelatin
2 tablespoons honey
1/8 teaspoon salt
3 egg yolks

1 1/4 cups fresh skim milk
1 teaspoon rum flavoring
1/4 teaspoon nutmeg
3 egg whites

Mix gelatin, honey, and salt in top of double boiler. Beat together egg yolks and skim milk. Add to gelatin mixture. Cook over boiling water, stirring constantly until gelatin is dissolved, about 5 minutes. Remove from heat, add rum flavoring and nutmeg. Chill until it thickens slightly. Beat egg whites until stiff and fold in gelatin mixture. Turn into molds and chill until firm. (Serves 6.)

Apple Yogurt Mousse
(About 60 calories per serving)

1 cup yogurt
2 cups applesauce
   (unsweetened)

1/4 teaspoon cinnamon
Fresh shredded coconut, for
   garnish

Blend yogurt with applesauce and cinnamon. Put into sherbet glasses. Garnish with fresh coconut before serving. (Serves 6.)

Low-Calorie Meringue Cakes
(About 34 calories per serving)

1 egg white
2 tablespoons powdered
   skim milk

1/4 teaspoon vanilla
1 tablespoon honey
Cinnamon

Beat egg white until it stands up in peaks, add skim milk powder. Continue beating until well mixed. Add vanilla and honey. Preheat oven to very hot temperature. Pour mixture into 4 compartments of muffin tin. Reduce heat. Bake at medium temperature until tops of cakes are round and evenly formed. To test, insert toothpick and if it pulls out clean, the meringue cakes are ready. Dust with cinnamon and serve. (Serves 4.)

Raspberry-Apricot Soufflé
(About 50 calories per serving)

3 egg whites
2 cups fresh or frozen raspberries
⅛ teaspoon cinnamon
⅛ teaspoon powdered ginger
6 apricot halves (fresh, frozen, or canned water-pack)

Beat egg whites until stiff peaks form. Fold in raspberries, cinnamon, and ginger. Divide among 6 sherbet glasses and garnish with apricot halves. (Serves 6.)

"Haven't you forgotten something?" you may ask. Have I? I promised you low-calorie desserts without sugar, and there they are, rich in the health-giving proteins of skim milk, eggs, and gelatin, with honey for added flavor as well as energy.

Still you're not satisfied? What's wrong?

It is true I said that you could have *one day*, once in a while, to forget about calories and eat whatever you pleased.

Is it pie you crave?

All right—why not?

There is a delicious, healthful, orange yogurt pie which is one of the exclusive delicacies served in a New York restaurant—*not* low in calories, but they *are* protein calories.

Here is a slightly modified recipe of the original rich version. It has the same haunting flavor, but cuts down a little on the calories.

Orange Yogurt Pie

1 envelope unflavored
   gelatin
¼ cup cold water
2 egg yolks
¼ cup fresh skim milk
1 cup (8 ounces) creamed
   cottage cheese

1 tablespoon honey
1 teaspoon grated orange
   rind
1 teaspoon vanilla
½ pint yogurt
Coconut Pie Shell
Orange sections

In top of double boiler, sprinkle gelatin over cold water to soften, then stir over hot water to dissolve. Beat egg yolks lightly, blend with milk, add to gelatin. Cook and stir constantly over gently boiling water until mixture coats a spoon. Remove from heat and cool. Cream the cheese, honey, grated orange rind, and vanilla. Gradually mix in yogurt, keeping smooth. Slowly stir in the cooled gelatin mixture and mix well. Chill until thickened, about 20 minutes. Beat until creamy and smooth, about 5 minutes. Pour into pie shell. Chill until firm. Before serving, garnish with orange sections. (Serves 8.)

Coconut Pie Shell

Mix unsweetened, finely ground coconut (sometimes sold as macaroon coconut), with 3 tablespoons safflower oil. Spread over bottom and sides of an 8-inch pie pan, making sides as thick as bottom. Bake in slow oven (325 degrees) 20 to 25 minutes. Cool before filling.

One of the really great actors of the American theater, Guy Bates Post, has kept his weight the same as it was when he played in one of his greatest successes, *The Masquerader,* back in 1917.

He and his lovely wife, the former Lady Lily Kemble-Cooper, usually prefer simple desserts of fruit or cheese, but here is the recipe for one of their favorite pies which they have on special occasions.

Luscious Lemon Cream Pie

3 egg yolks
1 tablespoon grated lemon rind
¼ cup honey
¼ cup lemon juice
3 egg whites
¼ teaspoon salt
¼ cup honey (yes, *again!*)
1 cup double-strength skim milk (use ¼ cup powdered skim milk mixed with cold water to make 1 cup)
¼ teaspoon vanilla
⅔ cup graham cracker crumbs

Mix egg yolk, lemon rind, and honey in saucepan. Gradually add lemon juice, stirring until smooth. Cook over low heat, stirring constantly until thickened, about 5 minutes. Beat egg whites with salt until they hold their shape. Continue beating and slowly drizzle in ¼ cup honey. Beat until meringue is stiff, then fold into warm mixture and let cool. Whip powdered skim milk and cold water until stiff. Add vanilla. Fold into cooked mixture. Sprinkle half of graham cracker crumbs over bottom of 8-inch pie pan or refrigerator freezer tray. Pour lemon cream over crumbs. Sprinkle top of pie with remainder of crumbs. Freeze until firm before serving. (Serves 6.)

Fresh fruit or berry pies are allowed weight-watchers once in a while on eat-for-a-treat days. But never, *never* any pie crusts made with white flour and lard, and never any top crust at all.

Make them open face, with honey for sweetening, if desired, and a bottom crust of crushed whole-wheat rusk, zwieback, or graham cracker crumbs moistened with enough safflower oil to hold them together.

Even then you'd be better off, calorie-wise, to eat the filling and leave the crust . . . *but just once in a while* . . . ? Oh, very well, go ahead and eat a few bites of it—I expect you would, anyway, wouldn't you?

But taste and savor, if you want to eat and *stay* slim. On the joyous day when your body is lithe again, and you feel lovely as can be, you'll swap your old feelings of doubt and insecurity for those of confidence and real joy in living.

You'll have traded weariness, illness, and discontent for energy, health, and happiness.

Don't ever trade back again!

16

How To Eat and Stay Slim

YOU'VE REDUCED, and you want to stay reduced. Never again will you start piling on unwanted pounds, if you can help it.

And you *can* help it.

You may need a little encouragement from time to time (who doesn't?) but you won't have to go very far to find it. Why not take a look at a few living examples who can provide enough incentive and inspiration to last the average person a lifetime?

Let's go behind the scenes and see how some famous figures stay as slim as they are.

When the Incomparable Hildegarde presented her one-woman show in Los Angeles recently, a producer who has known her for more than twenty years said, "That girl is incredible! She's still just as slender, youthful, and full of vitality as she was twenty years ago."

Just how does she do it? What's her secret?

"I eat carefully," Hildegarde says, "both to maintain my health and my figure. I like a healthy breakfast of two boiled eggs, fresh fruit in season, and sometimes a piece of whole-grain bread with soy spread and honey. I've learned to do without coffee, and I make my own mixture of herb tea by combining mint tea, rose hips, and fenugreek tea in small gauze bags. Sometimes I experiment with other combinations of herb teas for variety, and all are healthful and delicious."

Wherever she travels, part of Hildegarde's luggage is a big wicker basket which she calls her portable kitchen.

"I wouldn't be without my fruit-and-vegetable juicer," she says. "Every day I make a health cup of carrots, parsley, and dandelion greens or spinach. I always have my meat broiled or roasted, and my vegetables steamed. I've trained my appetite so that I don't get hungry for dessert, and never finish a meal with anything rich or heavy. If I want something sweet, fresh fruit, with its natural sugar, makes the perfect dessert."

Hildegarde's favorite salad is automatically served to her in the hotels where she has performed year after year. They have named it the Hildegarde Salad, in her honor, and she never tires of it.

The recipe is simple: water cress, romaine (or other lettuce), a shredded raw carrot, chopped parsley, and diced celery. The only dressing that she uses is the one which I recommend—*safflower oil mixed with a bit of lemon or lime juice.* Over this she sprinkles a generous handful of shelled sunflower seeds for an unusual flavor as well as for the added nutrition contained in the seeds in the form of protein, B vitamins, and vitamin A.

Hildegarde's other eat-to-stay-slim habits include one or more glasses a day of a freshly made raw vegetable vitamin vitalizer, plus daily multiple vitamin-and-mineral food supplement and alfalfa tablets.

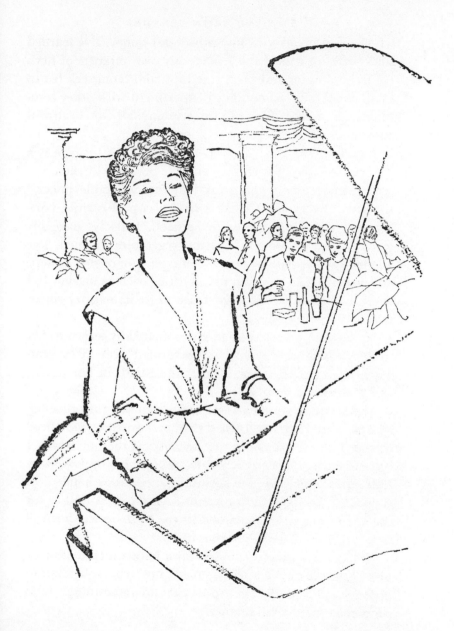

Whatever age Hildegarde is, it's a charming age which looks wonderful on her. Does she carry her own fountain of youth in that portable wicker-basket kitchen?

She says that she has trained herself to like only natural, wholesome foods. These include the proteins of broiled meat, chicken, fish, boiled or poached eggs, and cheese, the vitamin- and mineral-rich fresh fruits, raw vegetables, and juices, and lightly steamed vegetables.

By her own efforts—just as you can do!—she has consistently followed the rules of eating to stay slim, young, and vibrant.

Not too long ago the young, talented, and beautiful Mitzi Gaynor felt that she was a has-been. She was out of work and depressed because no good parts were coming her way. She turned to food for consolation, and started gaining weight until she had piled an appalling 150 pounds on her small bones.

"At that weight I was a fat-face," she says. "My eyes were scarcely visible in the folds of flesh around them. My future looked dismal, my clothes were dowdy—nothing but dowdy clothes would fit my forty-inch hips—and I'd have been completely desolate except for one man."

Her fiancé, Jack Bean, believed in her. (He's now her husband.) He had faith in her ability as an actress and in her potential as a person.

"Somehow he transmitted that faith to me," Mitzi says. "He encouraged me to go on a well-balanced, low-calorie diet, and I lost thirty-five pounds in three months. A whole new world opened up for me, and fabulous movie offers started coming my way, including that part which every actress wanted, Nellie Forbush in *South Pacific*."

Here is a sample of Mitzi's Take-Your-Choice diet:

BREAKFAST

½ grapefruit, 1 orange, or 4 ounces orange juice
2 eggs, soft-cooked or poached
Black coffee
(*No bread or toast.*)

LUNCH

½ small broiled chicken or 2 small lamb chops, fat
    trimmed off, or broiled chopped steak, or broiled steak
Fresh green or yellow vegetable
½ head lettuce or other green salad (with diet dressing
    or safflower oil and lemon juice)
Tea and nonfat milk

DINNER

Choice of the above selections, with an added dessert of
fresh fruit or a small portion of unsweetened applesauce.

Mitzi now weighs 115, and intends to stay that way. "I
took eight inches off my forty-inch hips," she says, "and
three inches off my waist. I'm concentrating on keeping a
firm contour of my face and body, so I do a neck exercise
every day. *And I don't have to diet any more. I can eat
and stay slim because I've learned to like the things that
are good for me.*" (Italics mine.)

Theodore Bikel, actor and singer, who played opposite
Mary Martin on Broadway in *The Sound of Music,* recently lost thirty pounds. His, too, was a high-protein
Take-Your-Choice diet of broiled meats, fresh green and
yellow vegetables, and choice of fruit for lunch and din-

ner. Breakfast was fairly standard, with eggs, fresh fruit or juice, black coffee and skim milk.

When he was asked if he ever cheated on his diet, Theodore said, "I never cheated on the forbidden foods such as bread, fats, or sweets. Sometimes when I was hungry I'd eat a larger portion of meat or vegetables and fruit."

Let him explain to you why he knows that from now on he'll be able to eat and stay reduced. "The old fat-making foods are just not as tempting as they used to be," he says.

Tom Donnelly used to be a big man in Washington. A popular columnist for the Washington *Daily News,* he loved to eat—and he ate himself up to a health-shattering 350 pounds.

Today he's still a big man in his profession, and he still loves to eat, but in less than a year he lost 175 pounds.

How did he do it?

He reduced the only safe, sure, and permanent way— on a high-protein, low-calorie diet, combined with the skillful art of substituting delicious, satisfying meals for the forbidden fat-making foods.

Donnelly doesn't like counting calories. (Lots of people don't, and they have the figures to prove it!) But he has an educated palate which stimulates him to creative efforts of substitution.

"Meat is the silver lining of the diet cloud," he says, "and I learned to brown meat without fat. Here's one of my favorite low-calorie gourmet dishes: Put some skim milk in a pan. Sprinkle lean veal chops with salt, cinnamon, and ginger. Put them in the pan and broil, basting occasionally."

Here is his original recipe for a low-calorie sauce for shrimps:

Blend (in an electric mixer) a fresh tomato or two with some fresh or dried basil, a twist of lemon peel, a little lemon juice, a sliver of garlic, and dashes of Worcestershire sauce and Tabasco. Add to this sauce some fresh chopped celery and celery leaves.

"I'd like to urge all fatties to spend their soda fountain money on meat," Donnelly says. "But if you're absolutely famished for a banana split, make it a low-calorie substitution, like this: On a banana half (50 calories) put a scoop of ice milk or water sherbet, and pour over it a sauce made of fresh strawberries or black cherries moistened with orange juice."

A diet doesn't have to be dreary. It can be a lifetime eating plan filled with imaginative, nonfattening substitutions and exciting experiments with food.

If you follow the eat-to-keep-fit slogan of the best athletic coaches, you'll have no trouble keeping your weight down. The foods which give you health and endurance keep you trim and firm as they condition you.

Australia's Percy Cerutty, called by some the greatest track coach the world has ever seen, has his training camp at Portsea, sixty miles down the coast from Melbourne. Six world records have come out of that camp, and among those who have trained there are the famous four-minute milers, John Landy, Murray Halberg, Albert Thomas, and Herb Elliott. John Landy was the second man to break the four-minute barrier in the mile race, and more recently, Herb Elliott reduced Landy's mile record of 3:58.0 to an amazing 3:54.5.

At the British Empire Games in 1958, Cerutty athletes won all of the long races from the half mile to the marathon. In Herb Elliott's four California appearances he broke that once unbreakable four-minute barrier three times.

These record-breaking feats happen too consistently to write them off as mere luck or coincidence.

How do Cerutty athletes train? *What do they eat?* When Herb Elliott was in America, he spent a few days at the home of Cordner Nelson, editor of *Track and Field News.* The runner's choice of breakfast seemed a little odd to his astonished host, but the cook must have loved it.

It's the same kind of breakfast that Swiss mountain climbers eat to give them endurance—a bowl of uncooked oats (Elliott mixes his with wheat germ), chopped nuts, dried figs, dates, and raisins, or other available fruit such as sliced bananas, peaches, or apples.

Less rugged individualists may soak their oats overnight in enough water to cover them. Cerutty athletes in Australia eat steel-cut oats, which haven't had all of the vitamins and minerals milled out of them. Steel-cut oats are available in this country in health food stores, and are one of the best sources of an all-around beauty mineral, silicon.

Silicon is essential for the growth of your hair and nails. It brightens your eyes, gives luster to your skin, and keeps it from becoming flabby. Silicon-rich foods included in your meals aid protein in fighting the flabbiness that dieters dread, and that we know now to be unnecessary.

"We eat as much raw, natural food as possible," says Cerutty. "For lunch we have a comprehensive salad consisting of almost anything—fresh fruit, raw vegetables chopped up with meat or fish, mild cheeses, hard-cooked eggs, and an oil dressing. Animal fats in any form are taboo: no butter, drippings, lards, or anything similar go into our food preparation. *Nothing but vegetable oil is used.*"

Dinner consists of rare roast or broiled meat, broiled poultry or fish, and lightly cooked vegetables in season. No potatoes except baked ones are served, and Cerutty says, "The vegetables are softened rather than cooked. The water they're steamed in is never thrown out—it's a valuable elixir."

All of these are suggestions that I've made to you repeatedly, but Cerutty's athletes are spectacular living examples which prove my point far better than words alone can do.

Jack La Lanne, television's most fervent advocate of eating and exercising to stay slim and fit, gives his audience a sound basic eating plan which is like the one that I have stressed for years.

"Correct eating is not staying on a hard diet," he says. "It's simply a matter of not overindulging, and of eating good, wholesome food in as much a natural state as possible. If you want to feel like a new person try eating just fresh fruit, eggs, and meat for a few days. And I'd like to see more people eating the inexpensive cuts of meat which are so good for all of us—hearts and kidneys, for example."

You think you don't like kidneys? Don't be too sure about it until you've tried them this way:

Slice a pound of prepared kidneys half an inch thick and cook them in ½ cup consommé and ½ cup tomato juice. Add ½ cup of sliced mushrooms, a clove of garlic on a toothpick, salt and pepper. Simmer for 20 minutes, remove garlic, and serve. (Serves 4.)

This makes a high-protein, iron-rich dish which is very low both in calories and cost.

By this time you've established a balanced, nutritionally sound way of eating. High in protein, vitamins, and minerals, and low—very low!—in fats and carbohydrates.

From now on it's up to you. You've been given the rules. You've seen how others have done it. You should be able to eat and *stay* slim simply by making a few small adjustments or substitutions in your eating habits.

Do you want some examples? All right.

Suppose that you're tempted to drink two glasses of whole milk a day, and you rationalize, "After all, milk is a complete protein—why shouldn't I drink all I want?"

I shouldn't have to tell you, but I will.

An eight-ounce glass of whole milk is loaded with 166 calories. Not just protein, but butterfat. By substituting buttermilk or fresh skim milk you can cut your calorie count in half. The number of calories saved on this substitution alone will give you a weight loss of approximately sixteen pounds in a year.

Maybe you like potatoes, but you've learned to limit yourself to one serving a week. An easy substitution allows you to eat that occasional potato and stay slim. Instead of hash-brown or French fries, have a baked potato topped with a spoonful of yogurt or cottage cheese and a sprinkle of chopped chives. Butter? You'll never even miss it. And you'll prevent a weight gain of four pounds a year. Four pounds may not sound like a lot, but remember that it goes into your calorie bank deposit, which is easy to save but hard to spend. The pounds can sneak up on you again before you know it. And sad to say, they don't sneak off you quite so easily.

Make moderation your watchword. By following a basic, well-balanced, eat-and-stay-slim plan you can allow yourself an eat-for-a-treat bonus now and then and still prevent that sneaky weight accumulation.

You may, as Theodore Bikel did, eat more meat, eggs, fruit, and vegetables, as hunger dictates. And of course you may eat practically all you want of the low-calorie raw vegetable slimming snacks listed in a previous chapter.

You *know* what to avoid in your eat-and-stay-slim plan: the fattening fifteen, the calorie bums.

You've lessened your food capacity and shrunk your stomach until your appetite is under control. You can keep it that way if you'll never again form the habit of eating the huge amounts of food you used to crave.

Don't deliberately overeat, even if your hostess urges second helpings. Never stuff yourself just to be sociable. Refuse to be an Alibi Annie or Freddie the Fall Guy.

They're the ones who whine that they can't eat and stay slim. But it's never their own fault. They always have an alibi for overeating. According to them, they never fall off the weight-control wagon. They're pushed, pushed by insistent hostesses, persuasive friends, and trapped by circumstances and environment. They *enjoy* being pushed into overeating, or they wouldn't push so easily. They would learn to resist pressure, graciously but firmly.

Keep a mental picture of the slender, vital person that you have become and want to remain, and you won't be tempted to increase your food capacity and enlarge your nice, flat stomach by going on uncontrolled high-calorie binges with built-in bulges.

Your subconscious mind is highly suggestible to orders, ideas, thoughts, and impressions, so never give it (or your conscious mind, either) a negative, unflattering picture of yourself.

Always put your best foot, face, and figure forward, and each day try to live, work, love, dream—and *eat*—as if you were exactly the person that you'd like to be.

What you eat literally becomes *you*, whether it's the

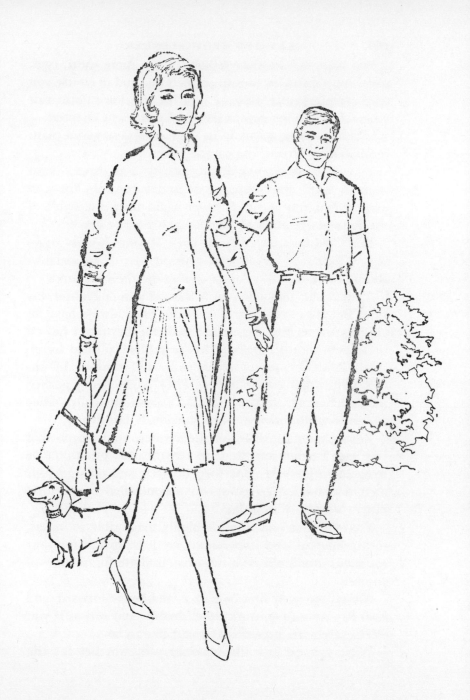

proteins, vitamins, and minerals that turn into healthy tissues, renewed cells, youthful skin, and a slim, firm body . . . or the calorie bums that become fat, sags, bags, and flabby droops of face, body, and spirit.

We know that it's a fact and not a theory that you *are* what you eat.

And remember, as humorist Fred Beck says:

"The more you eat the more you are."

Index

Abdomen, exercise for flattening, 124, 126, 131
Air bath, 74
Appestat, 87
Appetite, controlled by hypothalamus, 32
Appetite depressor, 59

Bacteria, friendly, 53
Banana split, in reducing diet, 58-59, 176
Banting, William, 72, 73
Basal metabolism rate, 66
Bean, Jack, 173
Beck, Fred, 183
Beef Stroganoff, low-calorie sauce for, 78
Bicycle exercise, 123, 126
Bikel, Theodore, 174-75, 180
Blackhall, Dotty, 64
Blood sugar, 75, 159, 210
Bouillon cubes, in reducing diet, 40, 50, 78
Boyle, Hal, reducing diet of, 84-85
Brady, William, 135
Bread, 51; lower-calorie, 51

Breakfast, importance of, 84, 97; in Shallcross diet, 83; in 900-1,000-calorie diet, 98-99; in 1,400-calorie diet, 88, 90
Brewer's yeast, 97
Brusch, Charles, 59
Bust - beautifying exercises, 131-32

Calcium, 74, 89
Calorie(s), in carbohydrates, 31; in cocktails, 44-45; in cottage cheese, 53; defined, 28; in desserts without sugar, 159-67; empty, 36-37; excess, stored as fat, 65; and exercise, 28, 30, 31, 65; in fats, 31, 71; in fruit juices, 115, 116; in fruits, 81; in high-carbohydrate fruits, 44; in honey, 208; in liquid diet drinks, 115-18, 119; in liquor, 44, 45; metabolic cost of digesting, 69, 70, 71; in milk, skim and whole, 179; need of, per pound of normal body weight, 28; in

185

Special Supplement

CONTENTS:

Chart Your Own Progress

Do you want to know how you're stacking up? (And I do mean literally.)

Then keep a record of your progress, not only in pounds but in inches. Fill in the form below. Read it and weep, if you must, or say, "M'mm, not bad. But it *could* be improved."

Here Are My Present Measurements:

Date_____

HEIGHT_____   BUST_____   THIGH_____

WEIGHT_____   WAIST_____   CALF_____

NECK_____   HIPS_____   ANKLE_____

WRIST_____   ARM_____

Yes, those measurements could be improved, couldn't they? And that's exactly what you're going to do. Let's leave a space for that, too.

Here Are My Future Measurements:

Date_____

HEIGHT_____   BUST_____   THIGH_____

WEIGHT_____   WAIST_____   CALF_____

NECK_____   HIPS_____   ANKLE_____

WRIST_____   ARM_____

Chart Your Own Progress

Do you want to know how you're stacking up? (And I do mean literally.)

Then keep a record of your progress, not only in pounds but in inches. Fill in the form below. Read it and weep, if you must, or say, "M'mm, not bad. But it *could* be improved."

Here Are My Present Measurements:

Date_____

HEIGHT_____   BUST_____   THIGH_____

WEIGHT_____   WAIST_____   CALF_____

NECK_____   HIPS_____   ANKLE_____

WRIST_____   ARM_____

Yes, those measurements could be improved, couldn't they? And that's exactly what you're going to do. Let's leave a space for that, too.

Here Are My Future *Measurements:*

Date_____

HEIGHT_____   BUST_____   THIGH_____

WEIGHT_____   WAIST_____   CALF_____

NECK_____   HIPS_____   ANKLE_____

WRIST_____   ARM_____

Chart Your Own Progress

Do you want to know how you're stacking up? (And I do mean literally.)

Then keep a record of your progress, not only in pounds but in inches. Fill in the form below. Read it and weep, if you must, or say, "M'mm, not bad. But it *could* be improved."

Here Are My Present Measurements:

Date_____

HEIGHT_____   BUST_____   THIGH_____

WEIGHT_____   WAIST_____   CALF_____

NECK_____   HIPS_____   ANKLE_____

WRIST_____   ARM_____

Yes, those measurements could be improved, couldn't they? And that's exactly what you're going to do. Let's leave a space for that, too.

Here Are My Future Measurements:

Date_____

HEIGHT_____   BUST_____   THIGH_____

WEIGHT_____   WAIST_____   CALF_____

NECK_____   HIPS_____   ANKLE_____

WRIST_____   ARM_____

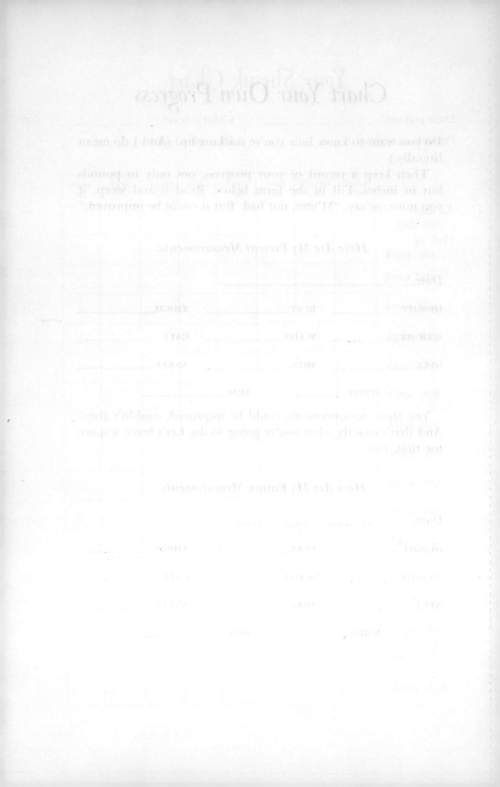

Your Shrink Chart

Date started_____   Calorie level_____

Pounds overweight_____   Desired weight_____

	weight lbs.	weight loss	bust in.	waist in.	hips in.	thighs in.	legs in.	arms in.
At start of diet								
End of 1st week								
2nd week								
3rd week								
4th week								
5th week								
6th week								
7th week								
8th week								
9th week								
10th week								
11th week								
12th week								
13th week								
14th week								
15th week								
16th week								

Your Shrink Chart

Date started_____   Calorie level_____

Pounds overweight_____   Desired weight_____

	weight lbs.	weight loss	bust in.	waist in.	hips in.	thighs in.	legs in.	arms in.
At start of diet								
End of 1st week								
2nd week								
3rd week								
4th week								
5th week								
6th week								
7th week								
8th week								
9th week								
10th week								
11th week								
12th week								
13th week								
14th week								
15th week								
16th week								

Your Shrink Chart

Date started_____   Calorie level_____

Pounds overweight_____   Desired weight_____

	weight lbs.	weight loss	bust in.	waist in.	hips in.	thighs in.	legs in.	arms in.
At start of diet								
End of 1st week								
2nd week								
3rd week								
4th week								
5th week								
6th week								
7th week								
8th week								
9th week								
10th week								
11th week								
12th week								
13th week								
14th week								
15th week								
16th week								

Your Cheat Chart

It's easy to chart your own progress if you know what rules you're breaking and how often you're cheating. Also where, when, and under what circumstances.

Then decide what you must do about it—and do it!

You might start by asking yourself these questions, and answering them honestly:

1. Have I sneaked a cooky or a piece of candy when nobody was looking? *Yes*_____ *No*_____

2. Have I substituted food for companionship and tried to kid myself into thinking that what nobody sees me eat won't make me fat? *Yes*_____ *No*_____

3. Have I dipped heavily into butter instead of using a low-calorie cottage cheese spread? *Yes*_____ *No*_____

4. Have I neglected my midday protein pick-up or vitamin vitalizer and gobbled up sugar and starch in the form of sweet rolls and doughnuts? *Yes*_____ *No*_____

5. Have I failed to do some exercise regularly so that I'll firm up as I shape up? *Yes*_____ *No*_____

6. Have I forgotten to do my face-firming routine to prevent sags and bags?   *Yes*_____ *No*_____

7. Have I eaten the fat on meat instead of trimming it off before cooking?   *Yes*_____ *No*_____

8. Have I been careless about taking a daily vitamin-mineral food supplement, even though I know how much it contributes to my health and well-being at any time, and especially when reducing?   *Yes*_____ *No*_____

9. Am I still using the frying pan for cooking?
          *Yes*_____ *No*_____

10. Have I eaten any of the fattening fifteen today?—yesterday?—or all week?   *Yes*_____ *No*_____

For a perfect score, all ten questions should be answered *no*. If you had a few *yes* answers, just allow a little margin for error and try harder tomorrow.

If you had all *no* answers, you're almost too good to be true—are you sure you weren't cheating on the cheat chart?

Is Your Diet Right for You?

1. Do you get a hungry, all-gone feeling soon after eating breakfast, lunch, or dinner?   Yes_____ No_____

2. Do you wake up tired, and are you tense, jittery, and irritable a good deal of the time?   Yes_____ No_____

3. Do you eat more starchy food than you do meat, leafy green and yellow vegetables, and fresh fruit?
     Yes_____ No_____

4. Are you susceptible to colds and sore throat?
     Yes_____ No_____

5. Do you suffer from frequent headaches or often feel weak and dizzy?   Yes_____ No_____

6. Are your skin and hair either excessively dry or oily?   Yes_____ No_____

7. Do you ever skip breakfast or have just coffee and toast?   Yes_____ No_____

8. Are you losing more than two pounds a week on your diet?   Yes_____ No_____

9. Does the skin on your hands and legs tend to become dry and flaky, or do your fingernails split and break easily?   *Yes*_____ *No*_____

10. Do you frequently neglect eating a protein food at each meal?   *Yes*_____ *No*_____

If you can honestly answer *no* to all of these questions, your diet is right for you. If you're not already slender, attractive, and full of vitality, you're well on your way.

Even *one* yes answer is a warning signal that your eating habits need changing. Try adding more meat, eggs, fresh vegetables and fruits to your menus, and take a daily vitamin-mineral food supplement to pull your diet out of the danger zone.

"Please Tell Me, Doctor..."

1. "When dieting should I cut out fats completely?"

No, indeed. Eliminate the hydrogenated fats (margarine, butter, lard, and other solid shortening), but even on a diet you need two or three teaspoons of unrefined vegetable oil each day, either mixed with lemon juice for a salad dressing or used as cooking oil. I particularly recommend *safflower oil* as a valuable source of essential fatty acids (polyunsaturates), vitamin E, and lecithin.

2. "Which supplies more iron in my diet—eggs or meat?"

The same amount by weight of eggs and the lean part of meat supply approximately the same amount of iron.

3. "Is calf's liver higher in food value than beef or lamb liver?"

No. All liver, including the cheaper beef or lamb liver, is a fine source of protein, iron, vitamins A, B complex, D, and E.

4. "Do all common foods furnish vitamins?"

No, not all. Refined white sugar, as one example, does not contain a single vitamin—only empty calories.

5. "I can lose several pounds by taking a steam bath, but I gain them back immediately, even without eating. Can you tell me why?"

Weight lost by perspiring, whether in a steam bath or by

violent exercise, is no more than a temporary loss of water from the body. When you drink several glasses of water the fluid is replaced and your weight is back where it was.

6. "You recommend honey in your diets, and I use it all the time—a five-pound can every two weeks—but I can't lose weight. Why is this?"

Of course, you can't! Honey is a healthful, energizing, concentrated sweet, rich in vitamins and minerals, but it *isn't* low in calories. One tablespoonful contains about 65 calories, and I advise it only in moderation for anyone, especially weight-watchers.

7. "How can I be sure to get all of the nutrients possible out of the food that I buy?"

Some vitamins, the B group and vitamin C, in particular, are soluble in water. Don't soak your vegetables before cooking. Steam them, if possible, or cook them very lightly in just enough water to cover them. Save the vitamin-rich water that they have cooked in for soup-making. Also save the tops of vegetables, such as beets, turnips, celery, and the outside leaves of cabbage, endive, and lettuce to make low-calorie, vitamin-and-mineral-rich broths.

8. "I never use any white flour. I bake three times a week, but all of my bread, pies, and cakes are made with whole-wheat flour. Still my whole family is overweight. What shall I do?"

Stop baking pies and cakes! Who gave you the idea that whole-wheat pastries and bread aren't fattening? Whether they are whole-wheat, white, rye, or whatever, pies, cakes, and bread are all fattening. Whole-grain bread may be used *in moderation* (one or two slices a day), but pastries must remain on the forbidden fattening fifteen list.

Do's and Don'ts for Dieters

DO—

1. *Eat wisely and moderately,* as though not only your weight but your very life depends on it—as indeed it may.

2. *Watch your calorie cost of living.* If you eat only a few nibbles—say 20 or 30 calories—more each day than your body requires to function well, you will slowly but surely in the course of years put on quite a hunk of weight. (Hunks varying from ten to twenty pounds—and all from a few extra nibbles!)

3. Avoid monotony by eating a variety of foods. Make your eat-and-stay-slim menus an adventure in good eating at low calorie cost.

4. Condition your appetite gradually, and set a definite goal with a reasonable length of time allowed to achieve your weight loss.

5. Eat slowly, chew well, and savor every morsel to get a feeling of satisfaction and satiety from smaller portions of food.

6. Have an orange, grapefruit, tomato, cantaloupe, strawberries, or raw cabbage every day to be sure you get your quota of vitamin C, which can't be stored in the body and must be replenished each day.

7. Cut down on salt (but don't cut it out entirely, unless a salt-free diet is advised for reasons of health) to avoid water retention in the tissues. Better yet, use sea salt or a salt substitute.

8. Eat regular meals and eat them at regular times. Skipping a meal results in a lowered blood sugar level, fatigue, and uncontrollable hunger which causes you to overload your stomach at the next meal.

9. Be sure to have some protein (meat, poultry, eggs, fish, cheese, yogurt, skim milk, or buttermilk) with each meal.

10. Remember what Benjamin Franklin said, "A full belly makes a dull brain." Eat lean meals to attain a lithe, vital body and an active brain.

11. Do limit your liquid intake to one cup at mealtime, but drink as much water or other calorie-free beverage as you like *between meals.*

12. Follow Alfred Hitchcock's advice and have dinner an hour earlier, if necessary, to avoid the cocktail hour.

DON'T—

1. Don't change your eating habits too much too soon. And don't neglect to fortify your diet with a good vitamin-mineral food supplement.

2. Weigh yourself every day. Weighing once a week at the same time and with the same amount of clothes on gives a more accurate proof of your progress, and avoids the discouraging day-by-day fluctuation of weight, which is often due to fluid balance.

3. Cheat on your diet. (Hey, wait a minute!—remember these are the DON'TS, so *don't* get any ideas. Maybe you'd better precede the following statements with your own mental *don't,* just as a reminder.) Never mind—to avoid confusion I'll do it for you.

4. *Don't* get discouraged. You can and will reduce—*if you don't cheat.*

5. Don't go on trick, faddy, or crash diets which can only result in a temporary weight loss (your body will be so starved nutritionally that you'll eat the pounds right back on again) at the expense of your health and looks.

6. Don't go on any diet less than 800 calories a day—and that only for short periods—unless supervised by an authority on nutrition to assure well-balanced meals.

7. Don't be tempted by bootleg cookies or whatever goodies that Mom, Grandma, and others who "just can't bear to see you go hungry" bake for you.

8. Don't eat when you're tense or overtired. Rest and relax for a while, and drink a cup of hot tea or bouillon to take the edge off your hunger.

9. Don't eat highly seasoned foods, as they stimulate the appetite.

10. Don't be discouraged if you can't lose several pounds immediately. Water will often displace fat temporarily. Give your fluid balance time to adjust, and a weight loss may come suddenly and dramatically.

11. Don't wash your food down with water or other beverage or it will take more to satisfy you.

12. Don't bore everybody with a blow-by-blow account of your diet, and don't be a diet martyr. You can enjoy gourmet dishes and eat-for-a-treat meals at a low calorie cost, so don't feel sorry for yourself.